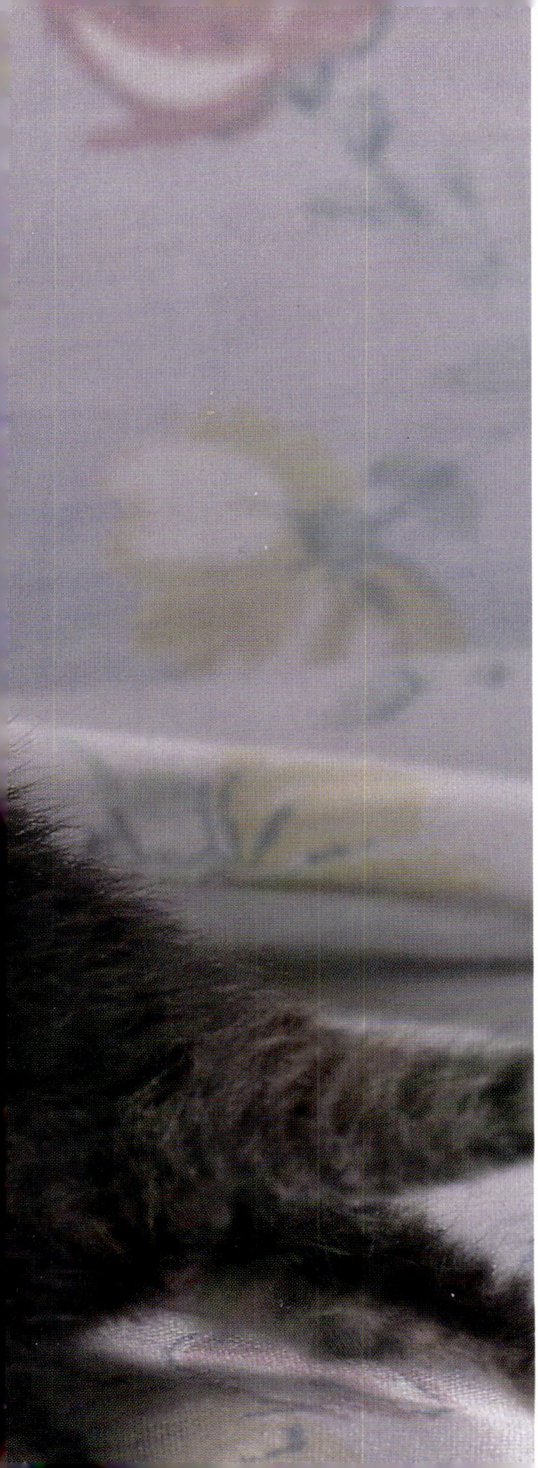

M. L. Papurt,

Hand-Raising the Orphaned Kitten

Filled with full-color photos

BARRON'S

Photo Credits

Norvia Behling: inside back cover, pages 2, 4, 6, 10, 15, 18, 23, 25, 33, 50, 51, 56, 60, 63, 67, 71, 76, 82, 84, 90, 91, 95; Susan Green: pages 24, 26, 29, 31, 34, 43, 45, 58, 59, 87; Bonnie Nance: back cover, pages 5, 8, 13, 21, 52, 54, 80, 89; The Stock Market Inc.: front cover, inside front cover.

About the Author

M. L. Papurt, DVM, is a graduate of The Ohio State University School of Veterinary Medicine and has been self-employed in the practice of veterinary medicine since 1962. She has written many newspaper and magazine articles concerning animal health issues. Other Barron's titles by Dr. Papurt include *Saved: A Guide to Success With Your Shelter Dog* and *Compatible Canines: Keeping the Peace Among Your Pets.*

All inquiries should be addressed to:
Barron's Educational Series, Inc.
250 Wireless Boulevard
Hauppauge, New York 11788
http://www.barronseduc.com

International Standard Book No. 0-7641-0727-5

Library of Congress Catalog Card No. 98-48069

Library of Congress Cataloging-in-Publication Data
Papurt, M. L. (Myrna L.)
Hand-raising the orphaned kitten / M.L. Papurt.
p. cm.
Includes bibliographical references and index.
ISBN 0-7641-0727-5 (pbk.)
1. Kittens. 2. Kittens—Diseases. I. Title.
SF447.P36 1999
636.8'089892—dc21 98-48069
CIP

Printed in Hong Kong

9 8 7 6 5 4 3 2 1

Important Note

When you handle cats, you may sometimes get scratched or bitten. If this happens, have a doctor treat the injuries immediately.

Make sure your cat receives all the necessary shots and dewormings, otherwise serious danger to the animal and to human health may arise. A few diseases and parasites can be communicated to humans. If your cat shows any signs of illness, you should definitely consult a veterinarian. If you are worried about your own health, see your doctor and tell him or her that you have cats.

Some people have allergic reactions to cats. If you think you might be allergic, see your doctor before you get a cat.

It is possible for a cat to cause damage to someone else's property and even to cause accidents. For your own protection you should make sure your insurance covers such eventualities, and you should definitely have liability insurance.

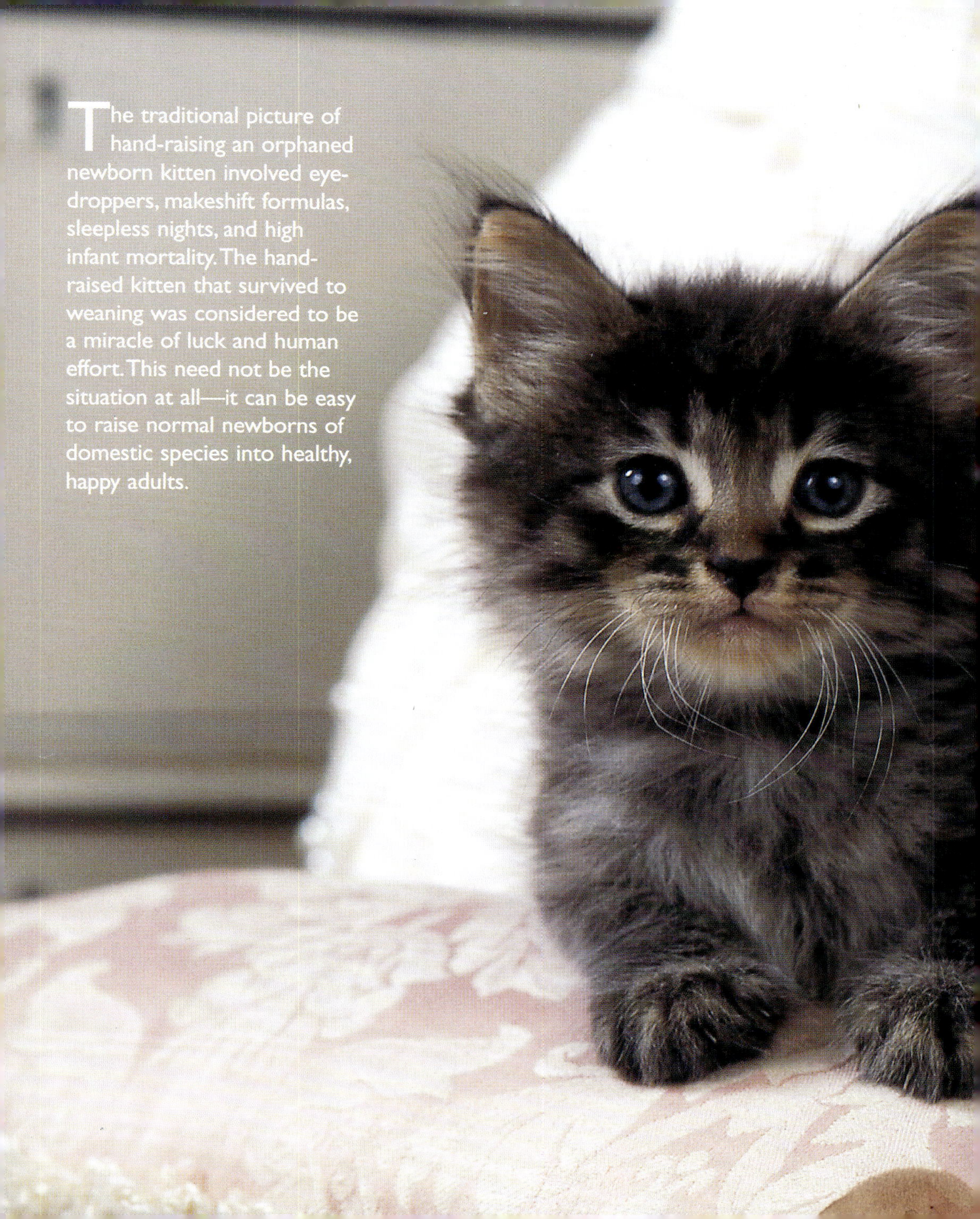

The traditional picture of hand-raising an orphaned newborn kitten involved eye-droppers, makeshift formulas, sleepless nights, and high infant mortality. The hand-raised kitten that survived to weaning was considered to be a miracle of luck and human effort. This need not be the situation at all—it can be easy to raise normal newborns of domestic species into healthy, happy adults.

Contents

Preface

Normal newborns of domestic species are surprisingly easy to raise. In spite of the fact that most infant mammals nurse a dozen or more times a day, these infants can survive and grow if fed far less frequently. Even though the exact composition of their dams' milk cannot be duplicated, orphans can and will thrive on formulas that only approximate what nature intends for them to have. Although maternal care can be best delivered by a mother animal, a human caretaker can provide sufficient warmth and sanitation to sustain orphans' lives.

You do not have to do everything perfectly to raise orphaned kittens to become perfectly normal cats. If you keep your orphans alive and growing reasonably well until they are able to eat by themselves, they will soon catch up to kittens raised by their own mothers. Your orphans may be smaller at weaning than if mother cats raised them, but they will not be stunted for life. Unless animals are maintained under conditions of starvation, they will eventually reach their genetically determined size.

Kittens raised by hand have the potential to become unusually loving pets. These kittens know no mother other than their human caretakers. They bond with humans with a strong, lifelong devotion. Hand-raised kittens trust humans to supply their needs. They consider humans to be the objects of their deepest affections. Hand-raising orphaned kittens is an emotionally rewarding experience.

When you undertake the chore of hand-raising orphaned kittens, you must realize that these kittens would not have survived without your efforts. When you cause them to survive, you accept the responsibility of ensuring that the kittens you save will not become part of the abandoned feral cat population.

Save those poor little orphans. When they grow into healthy kittens, keep them yourself or place them into responsible homes—homes that will have the kittens altered so the kittens cannot add to the population of feral animals.

If you cannot assume this responsibility, consider that not saving the kittens may be more humane. Do not raise kittens to love and trust humans only to have them abandoned to short, miserable lives of fear, hunger, and disease.

Chapter One

The Reproductive Cycle of the Domestic Cat

Cats Are Seasonally Polyestrous

The breeding season for domestic cats is normally the spring and summer months. From mid-autumn to early spring, most queens have no reproductive activity. The increasing length of daylight from January to March initiates feline breeding behavior. This is one of nature's survival tactics. Litters conceived in March are born in May when the weather is more conducive to kittens' survival. The breeding season for cats in Australia, where the seasons are the reverse of those in the United States, occurs during our winter months.

Cats are *seasonally polyestrous.* During the breeding season, each queen will have many (poly) heat periods (estrus). Each estrous period will average 5 to 15 days in length. A queen's estrous periods will occur at about two- to three-week intervals unless she becomes pregnant, is spayed, or the breeding season ends in the autumn. A great deal of variation occurs in the length of each estrous period as well as in the length between periods of each queen. To an owner, the queen will appear to be *in heat* on and off all spring and summer.

A healthy queen has no vaginal discharge during her estrous periods. She exhibits typical heat behavior of rolling, crying, posturing, urinating, arching her back, and treading with her hind feet. A few cats will have estrous periods at unusual times, which accounts for the litters of kittens occasionally born in the winter. Tomcats, of course, can and will breed all receptive females any month of the year.

The normal gestation period (length of pregnancy) for cats is 58 to 70 days, with an average of 63 to 65 days. An average litter consists of three to five kittens, although litters of eight or more are not uncommon.

The time of year, not the age of the female kitten, determines the start of the female's reproductive activity.

These kittens' eyes have just opened. They are still entirely dependent on their mother for food and care.

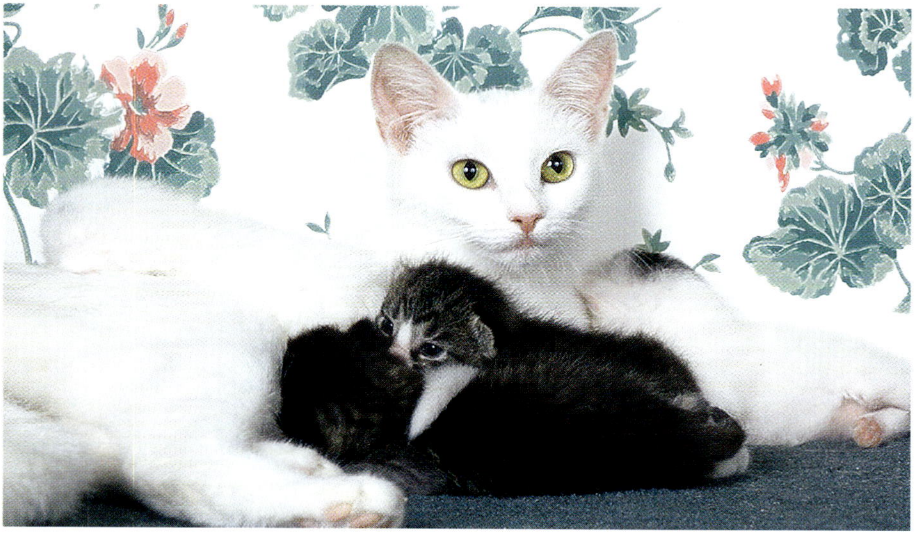

Female kittens born in the spring will have their first estrous period the following spring breeding season, when they are about nine or ten months of age. Female kittens born later in the summer will also have their first estrus near the beginning of the spring breeding season, although they may be only five or six months old. Owners of female kittens are advised to have them spayed in January or February of their first year. If the owners wait any longer, their kittens will go into heat.

Normal Development of Queen-Raised Kittens

The development of kittens raised by their mothers follows a typical pattern. This pattern depends on early protection against disease, birth weight, and weight gain.

Early Protection Against Disease

Antibodies are substances in an animal's blood that help protect it from disease. In some mammals, notably humans, antibodies in the mother's bloodstream enter the fetus through the placenta. The newborn child is born with some of its mother's immunity. In cats, most of the mother's antibodies do not cross into the kittens from the placenta. At birth, kittens have very few *maternally derived antibodies.*

Kittens receive antibodies when they consume *colostrum,* the first milk produced by their mothers. Colostrum contains antibodies from the mother's bloodstream for only 24 hours. The antibody content of a queen's colostrum gradually declines.

It is highest immediately after she gives birth and almost zero 24 hours later. Kittens are able to absorb these antibodies only until they are 12 to 24 hours old. Kittens must nurse within an hour or two of their birth to ensure that they receive as much maternally derived protection as possible.

Kittens that do not nurse before they are 12 hours old will have only 10 to 20 percent as much maternally derived immunity as those that received colostrum during the first 12 to 24 hours of their lives. Kittens that do not nurse during this critical time period will be at increased risk for bacterial and viral disease.

You must take extra precautions to raise colostrum-deprived kittens to weaning.

- Keep their beds and feeding equipment very clean. You must prevent bacterial contamination. Colostrum-deprived kittens will succumb to bacterial disease that would not affect kittens with adequate maternal antibodies.
- You must prohibit exposure to other cats. Colostrum-deprived kittens will have few antibodies to protect them from diseases carried by other cats.
- Handlers of colostrum-deprived kittens must remember to wash their hands between handling each member of the litter and to use very clean feeding equipment for each kitten.
- Kittens that were deprived of maternal antibodies will be receptive to vaccination at a younger age than kittens that received colostrum. Your veterinarian may recommend a different vaccination schedule for these kittens.

Normal Birth Weights Vary

Factors that influence the birth weight of kittens include the age and nutritional state of the queen, the number of kittens in the litter, and the length of gestation. On average, each kitten of a litter of four or five kittens, born after a 65-day gestation, will weigh between 3 and 5 ounces (75 to 125 g). If the kittens are born to a well-nourished mother after a 68- to 70-day gestation, each will weigh about 5½ to 6 ounces (100 to 150 g). The weight of each kitten will decrease slightly immediately after birth; this is caused by fluid loss of the newborn.

Kittens born after a longer gestation are usually better developed and heavier than those born after a short gestation. The eyes of kittens born after a long gestation will open correspondingly sooner than those born after a normal gestation of 63 to 65 days. The eyes of long-gestation kittens commonly open at five days in contrast with those of normal kittens that open at seven to ten days of age.

Normal Weight Gain of Queen-Raised Kittens

Weight gain in kittens depends on many factors, including the initial vigor of the newborns, the milk production of the queen, and the number of kittens in the litter. Under optimum conditions, gains of 2 to 4 ounces (50 to 100 g) a week are not

At three weeks, the kittens are starting to walk around.

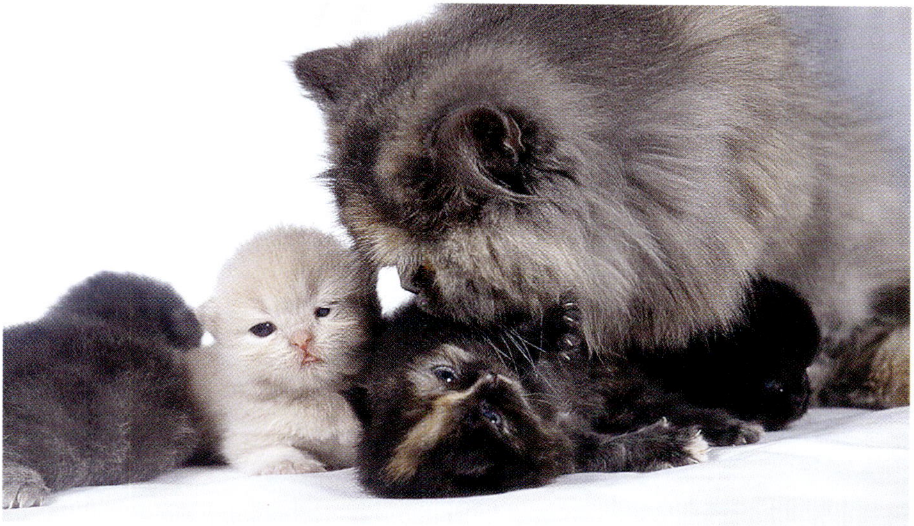

uncommon. At seven days of age, a kitten may weigh almost twice as much as it did at birth.

Inadequately nourished queens cannot produce sufficient milk to promote rapid gains in their kittens. Kittens born in large litters will receive a correspondingly smaller amount of milk. Kittens born to undernourished or parasitized queens may grow much more slowly or fail to thrive at all. So many variable factors influence neonatal kittens that adequate growth and optimum growth may differ greatly.

Kittens raised by their mothers will weigh approximately 14 to 18 ounces (400 to 500 g) at normal weaning, about six weeks of age. Males tend to weigh more than females, a difference that becomes more pronounced as the kittens grow older.

Do not worry if your hand-raised kittens are small. They will grow very rapidly when they start to eat solid food.

Expected Development of Hand-Raised Kittens

Nature has designed the milk of a mother cat to be the perfect food for her offspring. A queen nurses her litter for about 20 hours a day. Each of her kittens has an almost unlimited opportunity to feed whenever it feels hungry. A healthy and well-nourished queen produces milk on a continuous basis. Each kitten nurses a small amount more than ten times in every 24-hour period.

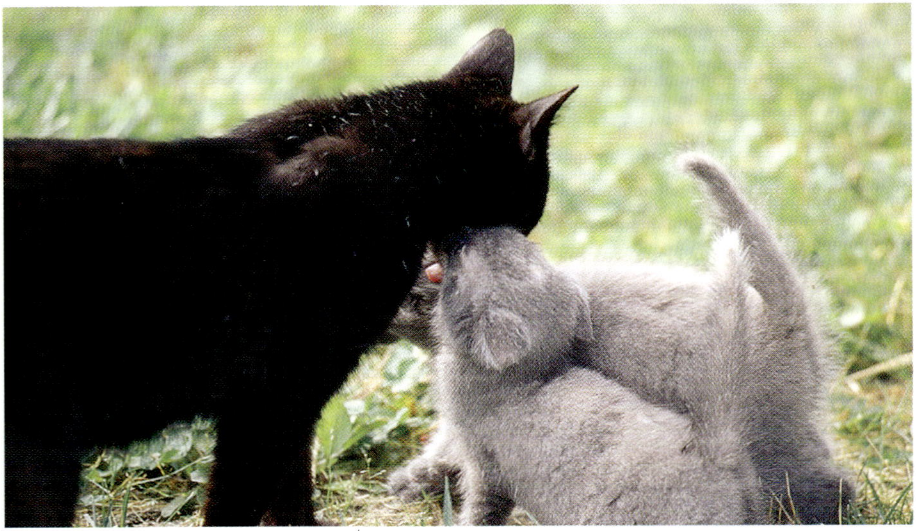

Five-week-old kittens are ready to be independent.

A hand-raised kitten is fed a milk substitute formulated by humans. The hand-raised kitten is given the opportunity to consume this milk only at specified times, often only four times in 24 hours. The hand-raised kitten receives only that volume of milk provided by its human handlers. If the hand-raised kitten is fed by a stomach tube instead of a nursing bottle, it does not even have control of the volume of milk it consumes. For these reasons, people should not wonder that hand-raised kittens will often lag behind queen-raised kittens in weight gains.

Rapid gain in weight is not the objective in hand-raising kittens. The object is to keep the kittens alive and developing at an acceptable rate until they are old enough to consume and digest solid food. Fortunately, hand-raised kittens can be weaned at four to five weeks. When kittens can eat by themselves, you can offer them nutritious food many times a day. The hand-raised kitten that weighs only 11 ounces (300 g) at weaning will catch up to the 18-ounce (500-g) queen-raised kitten by the time they are both three months old.

Chapter Two

When Hand-Raising Is the Correct Option

The Humane Society of the United States estimates that 40 percent of all kittens and puppies die before they are weaned. This means that four out of ten kittens do not live to reach five or six weeks of age.

This figure seems extremely high to pet owners. If *our* animals have babies, we make every effort to ensure that each one grows up healthy. We consider it to be a tragedy if even one kitten is lost. However, a huge number of kittens are born to cats that have no real owners. Many are born to cats whose owners are disinterested in their pets' welfare. These people hardly notice if Tabby has had another litter or if her kittens survive.

Occasionally, orphaned kittens can be valuable purebreds. Hand-raising purebred kittens is done to avoid an economic loss. Much more often, people raise orphaned kittens out of sympathy—it seems so cruel to allow these tiny bits of life to expire because their mother cannot raise them. Kittens may become orphaned for several reasons.

A tiny kitten depends on you for everything.

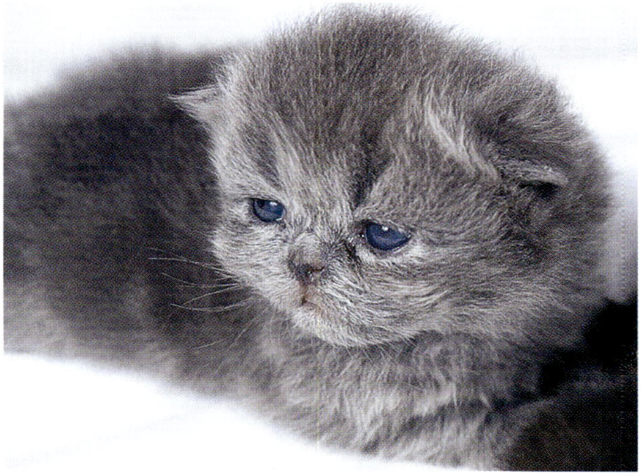

Maternal Death or Abandonment

The most common reason kittens become orphaned is the loss of the mother cat. The mother may die from complications of pregnancy or parturition. She may leave her brood for a few minutes and be hit by a car. She may be killed by a passing dog. She may simply disappear, leaving a hungry litter in the nest.

Cats are very efficient at reproduction. Deadly complications of pregnancy seldom occur in cats. Few feline pregnancies result in septicemia (infection) or dystocia (difficulty or inability to give birth). If queens with these problems are purebreds or valued pets, they usually receive veterinary care. If they are free-roaming or ignored outdoor cats, they often die unattended. In either case, a litter of kittens is left motherless.

Maternal Agalactia

Agalactia means without milk. Several factors influence the ability of a queen to produce enough milk for her kittens:

Starvation or Near-Starvation of the Queen. A queen nursing four to six kittens requires 150 to 300 percent more food than does a cat that is not nursing. The nursing queen also requires more high-quality protein in her diet if she is not to use up her body tissues to produce milk for her kittens.

A cat that is not being fed properly by humans or a cat that cannot successfully find her own food will use her body fat for energy to produce milk. When her fat reserves are depleted, her milk production will diminish. Eventually, her milk production will stop completely. An unfed cat that is very thin when she gives birth to her litter will be unable to produce milk until her kittens are old enough to wean. A starving cat may not produce enough milk to support her litter for even a week.

Mammary Gland Inflammation. Mastitis, an inflammation of the mammary glands, occurs occasionally in queens. Staphylococcal and streptococcal bacteria cause infectious mastitis. This may result in abscesses of the glands. The last pair of mammary glands (closest to the hind legs) are most often affected. Usually, the rest of the mammary glands are normal. However, the infection can make the queen too sick to produce milk or to care for her kittens.

Most queens recover from mastitis when they are treated with broad-spectrum antibiotics. The treatment, which requires at least two weeks, will not enable the cats to recover in time to raise their kittens. The kittens of a queen suffering from mastitis must be hand-fed if they are to survive. Such kittens should also receive antibiotic therapy for five to ten days.

Mammary Gland Tumors. Breast cancer in cats is uncommon, but it does occur. Most affected cats are seven years of age or older. Malignant mammary tumors in cats are usually adenocarcinomas. They grow and spread very rapidly and are often fatal to the queen. A pregnant queen that has mammary cancer seldom lives long enough to deliver and raise her kittens.

Lactation Tetany or Hypocalcemia. Hypocalcemia is also called *milk fever*. Depletion of calcium reserves from a queen's body causes

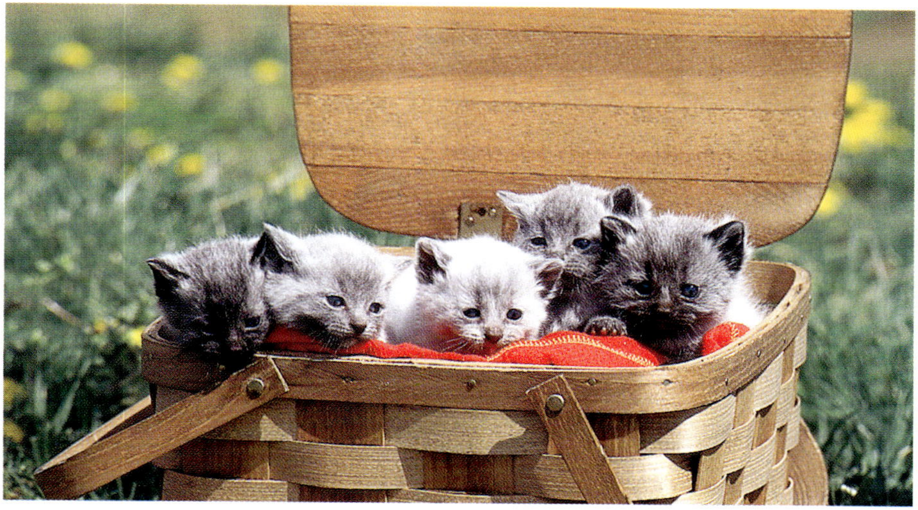

A large litter requires a lot of care.

this condition. Calcium is involved in the normal function of the nervous system. Low blood calcium may result in tremors, incoordination, convulsions, and death of the mother cat.

Hypocalcemia can occur in a queen with a large litter when she is producing a huge amount of milk for her three-to-four-week-old kittens. Hypocalcemia can be controlled by removal of the kittens, which will stop the queen's milk production. The queen should be treated with intravenous calcium. The kittens then must be hand-fed.

Maternal Aggression Toward Kittens

Most queens take very good care of their newborns: cleaning them, encouraging them to nurse soon after the kittens are born, and stimulating them to eliminate. A few first-litter queens, especially those that are very timid or are disturbed by a new environment, may ignore their kittens or actually act afraid or hostile toward them. Most of the queens with this behavior will accept their kittens in an hour or two if undisturbed in dark, quiet surroundings.

If a queen shows no maternal behavior four hours after the birth, her kittens should be removed and hand-raised. A longer wait may result in kittens that are chilled, starved, or actually attacked by their mother.

The Large Litter

The average litter size in domestic cats is four to six kittens. Seven or eight are not uncommon; some young queens may have only two or three kittens in their first litter. New-

born kittens should be left with their mother to obtain much-needed colostrum, or first milk, which contains antibodies important to kittens' health.

By the time the kittens are two to four weeks old, queens with seven or more kittens (or queens that are in very poor condition when they give birth) often cannot produce enough milk for their entire litter. If the kittens do not receive extra food, they may live but grow poorly. The weaker kittens may die.

Removing kittens from a queen that cares for them, even if her milk is insufficient for the litter, is not necessary or desirable. The queen can keep her kittens clean and warm. The human caretaker should offer each kitten formula from a bottle three or four times a day to supplement the mother's milk supply.

- Select a formula that the kittens can digest.
- Teach the kittens to drink from a bottle.
- Offer the formula to each kitten, not just the smallest ones.
- Kittens that are receiving supplemental feedings while they are nursing should be fed with a bottle, not a stomach tube. This will allow each kitten to consume only as much milk as it wants. If fed with a stomach tube, the kittens that are nursing adequately will be forced to consume too much milk. They might get diarrhea from overfeeding.
- If the kittens in a litter all look alike, identify them in some way to assure that each one has been fed.
- Kittens in litters receiving supplemental feedings should be offered solid food by the time they are four weeks old. They should be weaned by five weeks of age.

The Foster Mother

The easiest and often the most successful way to raise orphaned kittens is to let a foster mother cat do it. If you can find a queen in the appropriate stage of lactation and if you can convince her that the orphans are really her babies, she will do the work for you. She will do a better job than you possibly can since nature has equipped her for the task.

Finding a Foster Queen

Finding a foster mother for your orphans can be difficult. You must locate a queen that has kittens of approximately the same age as your orphans. You need a queen that has only a few kittens. If you have several orphans, you might need more than one nursing queen; that way you can foster one or two of your orphans on each queen.

You can use a queen whose kittens have died if the kittens did not die from a condition that could affect your orphans. Only occasionally can you persuade a queen that has recently weaned a litter to accept another batch of babies to raise.

Start your search for a foster queen by checking your local telephone directory. First look under

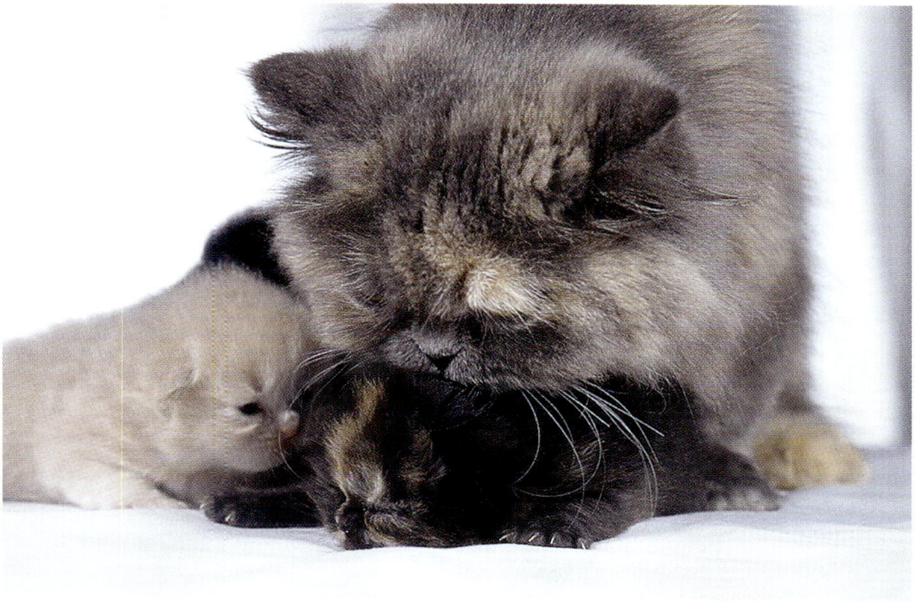

The queen cleans these two-week-old kittens very carefully.

"Humane Societies," then "Animal Wardens," then "Cats" or "Catteries." Call each number and explain your problem. You are much more likely to find a queen with a new litter at a humane society than at either of the other types of organizations.

Finding a Healthy Queen

The queen with kittens at an animal shelter is there because nobody wanted her. She has probably never received vaccinations against contagious feline diseases, treatment for parasites, or adequate nutrition. She may be covered with fleas, full of worms, or half-starved.

Once admitted to a shelter, the queen becomes exposed to other cats and the diseases they carry. Many shelters vaccinate their new animals. However, if vaccines are not administered before disease organisms proliferate in the queen's body, she will not be protected. Even though she becomes vaccinated, she may get sick.

Some shelters also treat their animals for internal and external parasites. You may be able to find a queen that is harboring few fleas or worms. If she does have these parasites, you can eliminate them by yourself or with the help of your veterinarian.

The most common diseases contracted by cats at a shelter are those that affect the cats' respiratory systems. Noses dripping mucus, sneezing, and thick discharges from the eyes are the usual signs. Really sick cats stop eating; a few will die.

If you adopt an apparently healthy queen from a shelter, you always take the chance that her body is incubating one of these diseases. If she is, she will show signs of illness within seven to ten days. Most sick cats from shelters have conditions caused by viruses. Antibiotics cannot cure these conditions.

If the queen is sick, her kittens will be affected. If you give her orphaned kittens to foster, the orphans will become affected. The sick queen may be able to raise the kittens. She will probably recover from the disease. However, her kittens and the orphans may develop signs of disease.

Fostering orphaned kittens on a nursing queen is much easier than hand-raising them on bottles. You must make the decision. Either risk acquiring a possibly sick queen or hand-raise the orphans.

If you decide to take a queen from a shelter, try to get one that appears to be free of eye and nose discharges. The shorter the time the queen was at a shelter, the greater her chances of being free of disease. However, her body may be incubating a virus that will become apparent a few days later.

If you have other cats at home and you get a shelter queen, keep her, her own kittens, and her foster kittens in a room by themselves. Prohibit contact with your other cats even if they have received vaccinations. Ask your veterinarian if you should get booster shots for your resident cats.

Use separate dishes and utensils to care for the new and the resident animals. Wash your hands before and after handling either group. Many feline respiratory viruses are airborne; keep the door closed between the two groups.

Persuading the Queen to Accept Orphaned Kittens

If you locate a queen with a litter close to the age of your orphans, go to the shelter and adopt her and her kittens. Place the queen and her litter into a big cardboard box with a cover. Line the box with the bedding from the humane society. The bed will smell the same to the mother cat. Cover the box for the trip home. Make sure the lid has airholes.

When you get the queen and her litter home, remove only the queen from the box. Close her in a cage or in another room where she cannot hear or smell her kittens. Give her some canned cat food and a bowl of water.

Place your orphans in the box with the queen's own litter. After an hour of crawling over each other, the orphans will smell very much like the queen's kittens, and the queen will be eager to be back with her litter. Allow her back with the kittens, but watch carefully. A few queens will detect your deception and will hiss at or actually attack the strange babies. If she does, take her away from the kittens for another hour, and try again to get her to accept the whole brood.

Do not allow the kittens to go without nursing for more than two or

three hours. If the queen will not accept the strange kittens, take them out and hand-feed them. Allow the queen to nurse her own litter. Sneak the orphaned kittens back in among the others, one at a time, over the next few hours. If all the kittens are nearly the same size and you are persistent, you will probably be successful.

Unless both the queen's litter and the orphans are less than two days old, your orphans will not receive colostrum, the antibody-rich first milk. They must receive the same extra attention as colostrum-deprived orphans that are entirely hand-raised.

If you locate a queen with a litter that you do not have to adopt from a shelter, do not disturb her nest box. Merely remove the queen for an hour or two. Place the orphans among her own kittens, and allow them to mingle and acquire each other's scent. When you allow the queen to return, she will probably accept the orphans as her own. Cats cannot count very well.

The Foster Mother with a Large Litter

If the only queen you can locate has a normal litter of four or five kittens and you have four or five orphans, you can still use her to raise the orphans. You will have to help her. The queen will be able to clean the kittens and keep them warm. However, she may be incapable of producing a large enough volume of milk to nourish more than five or six.

- Feed the queen all the good-quality canned cat food she will eat. Feed her four times a day. Canned food is very palatable. The mother cat will eat an enormous amount and use the nutrients and the moisture in the food to produce more milk.
- Many cat breeders supplement their queens' diets with a high-quality kitten food. Their queens use the extra energy content of kitten food to support lactation.
- Be sure the queen has an adequate supply of fresh water to drink. Do not worry if she seems to drink only a little; canned food contains at least 85 percent moisture. She may be getting most of the water she needs in her food.
- If the queen now has more than six kittens, place a heating pad turned to low under one end of the nest box. This will provide warmth in case all the kittens cannot get close enough to the queen. Electric heating pads must always be placed *underneath* the box, never inside the box. A kitten that crawls under the bedding and lies on an unprotected heating pad very quickly becomes dangerously overheated and may actually be burned. Even when the heating pad is turned to low, place towels or other insulation between the heating pad and the box to maintain the proper temperature.
- Prevent the weaker kittens from dying of starvation. A queen nursing seven or eight (or more) kittens will probably not be able to produce enough milk for each of the kittens

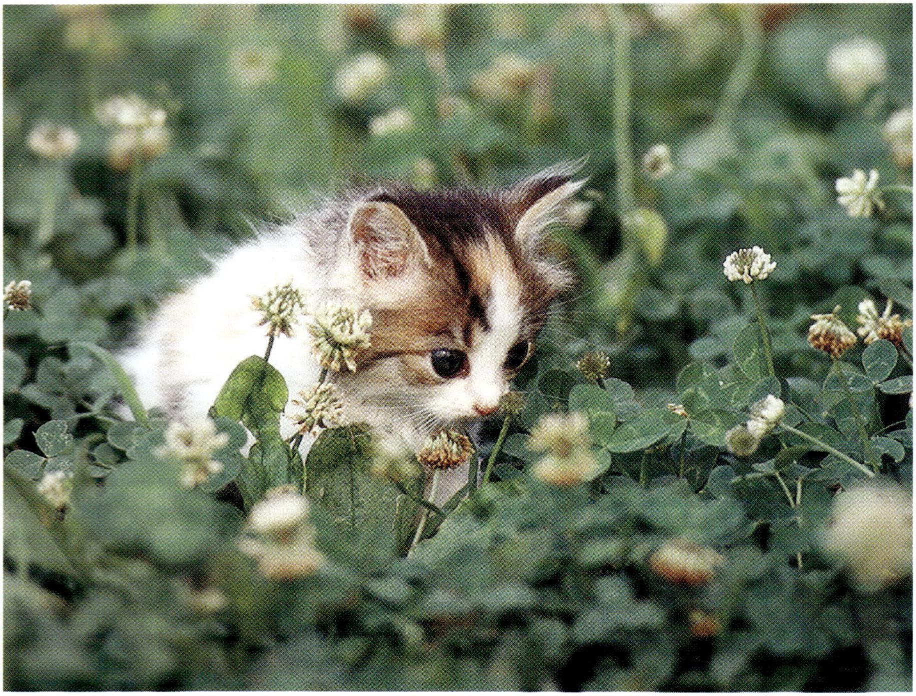

This kitten's name is Violet.

to thrive. Some of the kittens will be shoved aside by their littermates and foster littermates. Ultimately, the weaker kittens will become weaker still. Without help, some of the kittens may die.

Prepare a milk replacement formula and offer it to each kitten at least once every eight hours. The hungry kittens will drink. The ones nursing an adequate amount may refuse the bottle.

You may need to offer the formula to the weaker kittens more often than every eight hours. If the smaller kittens are frequently pushed aside, you may have to remove them and completely hand-feed them.

Identifying Each Kitten

You should keep a record of the weight gains and special problems of each individual kitten, so telling them apart is important. If your kittens are alike in color and size, you should mark them for positive identification.

Divide the litter into males and females. Even in newborn kittens, the difference between the sexes is not difficult to see. In females, the anal opening and the genital opening (vulva) are close together. In males, the anus and the opening of the penis are separated by a noticeable space of fur-bearing skin, the

scrotum. This will contain the male kittens' testes when the kittens are a little older. If you compare your kittens, the difference will be obvious. You will have difficulty telling males from females only if all the kittens are of one sex. A rule of thumb: if you cannot tell the sex, the kitten is probably a female.

When you prepare your records, give each kitten a letter for its sex and an individual number. For example, M-1 for male number one, F-1 for female number one, and so on. Next to each kitten's letter and number, describe the color and markings: M-1, black, white chest; M-2, all black; and so forth.

Kittens identical in color and sex must be marked to tell them apart. If the kittens are entirely hand-raised, they will be kept in separate beds until they are weaned. Their enclosures can be numbered and each kitten always returned to the same location. For weaned or fostered kittens, each must receive an identifying mark.

Marking kittens on their backs with ink, paint, or nail polish is possible once they are weaned. However, if nursing kittens have a foster mother, she will try to lick off the markings. A better method of marking individual kittens is to snip off a small spot of hair off their necks, shoulders, or backs. M-1 could be the male with a snipped spot on his neck; M-2, the male with a snipped spot over his shoulders; and so on. Of course, the hair will grow back, and you will have to snip it again at two-week intervals.

Emergencies

Healthy kittens feel warm and squirmy. They appear plump and have good skin tone. Healthy kittens try to remain in a crawling or nursing position on their stomachs and quickly regain that position if placed on their backs or sides. Healthy kittens usually stay together in a nest box. Healthy kittens may cry when picked up but seldom make a sound when not disturbed. When given the opportunity to nurse from a queen or a bottle, healthy kittens suck vigorously.

Sick kittens feel cold, thin, and limp. They lie scattered about the box. They may lie on their sides. They may cry weakly or incessantly for no apparent reason. Sick kittens are too weak to nurse.

Three common conditions cause sick, failing kittens: chilling, starvation and dehydration, and bacterial or viral disease (see Chapter 9 for information on diseases). The signs of each of the conditions are very similar. If you are confronted with failing kittens, do not try to make a diagnosis. The emergency procedures for all of the conditions are the same.

Chilling

Newborn kittens have not yet developed the ability to regulate their own body temperatures. Their mother keeps them warm with heat from her body. Kittens need their mother's warmth or supplemental heat until they are at least three weeks of age.

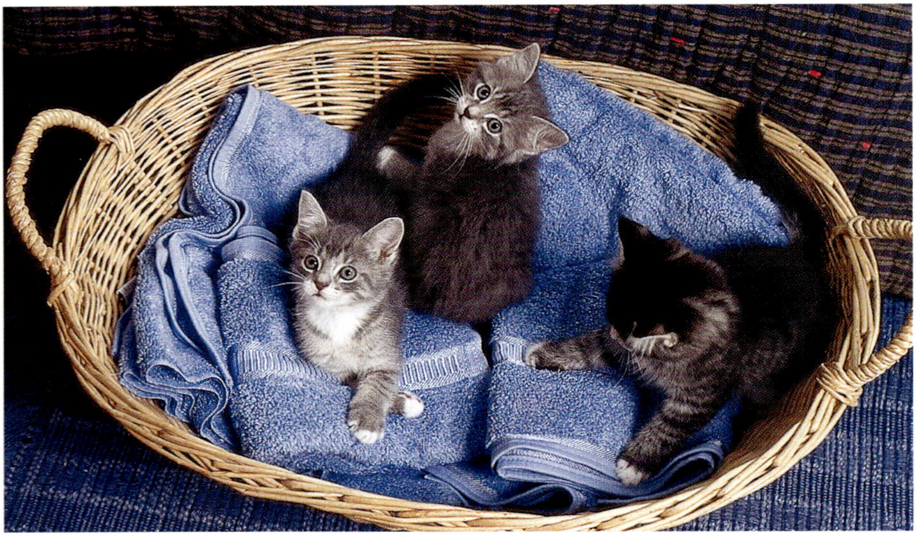

A basket full of healthy, hand-raised kittens.

A nursing queen's body temperature is about 102°F (38.9°C). This is the temperature to which the kittens should be warmed. Place the kittens onto an electric heating pad turned on low and insulated with towels to maintain a temperature of 101 to 103°F (38 to 39°C). If the kittens are merely cool, the pad will bring them to an acceptable temperature within 30 minutes. If the kittens are inactive, turn them every five minutes so their bodies warm uniformly. Do not allow the pad to become hot. The purpose is to warm the kittens, not to cook them. Do not leave kittens unattended on a heating pad unless the pad is *underneath* their box. Take absolutely no chance that a kitten could crawl under the bedding and be burned.

People often find orphaned kittens abandoned and thoroughly chilled. Such kittens must be warmed promptly if they are to have any chance to survive. Immersing chilled kittens up to their necks in warm running water will help heat their entire bodies. If the water feels the least bit hot to the human hand, it is too warm for kittens. Use a thermometer, and keep the water temperature around 102 or 103°F (38.9 to 39°C). Once the chilled kittens feel warm (after two or three minutes), dry them carefully, and place them onto an electric heating pad. Change their damp bedding frequently until the kittens are completely dry.

Chilling is a very serious condition in kittens less than a week old. The effects of severe chilling include increasing the kittens' susceptibility to bacterial infection of their intestinal and respiratory systems. Many chilled kittens survive only a few days.

Starvation and Dehydration

Starvation and dehydration almost always occur together. *Hypoglycemia* (low blood sugar) will kill kittens very quickly. Do not wait until they are warm and dry to get to a veterinarian for replacement of the kittens' body fluids and blood sugar. Get them as warm as possible, place them onto a warm hot-water bottle, cover their box with a towel to keep them warm, and drive to the nearest animal hospital.

When confronted with dehydrated and starving kittens, a veterinarian will administer a solution of 5 percent *dextrose* (a simple sugar) and *saline* (a weak salt solution). A normal newborn kitten weighs about 4 ounces (100 g). A veterinarian would give it about 0.3 ounces (5 ml) of the warmed solution subcutaneously (under the skin) or orally (by mouth) with a stomach tube. Once the veterinarian has instituted fluid therapy, he or she will explain to you how to continue treating the kittens at home.

Emergency Home Care

In many instances, rushing the kittens to a veterinarian is not a possibility. You might acquire the kittens in the middle of the night. You might be a long way from the nearest animal hospital. Let's face it. You may be unable or unwilling to spend a lot of money on kittens that might not survive, but you still intend to do the best you can to help them. What can you do at home in an emergency?

Homemade sugar solutions are for emergencies only. These formulas cannot replace veterinary care!

Kittens with hypoglycemia and dehydration must receive fluid replacements *immediately*, not milk, not even kitten formula milk. Milk and milk products must be digested by the kitten in order to enter its bloodstream. Dying kittens cannot wait; they need quick blood sugar replacement if they are to recover. They must have their fluid balance restored to normal as quickly as possible.

Ordinary granulated sugar is composed of *sucrose.* Sucrose is not a *simple sugar.* It must be digested before it enters the bloodstream. Therefore, a solution of table sugar cannot help your failing kittens. White corn syrup (Karo) is a simple sugar. In an emergency, you can use that. Commercial pancake syrup contains corn syrup plus sucrose, maple sugar, coloring, flavoring, preservatives, and other substances. Pancake syrup cannot be recommended for kittens. If you have no white corn syrup, a grocery store nearby probably has a bottle of it on the shelf.

In an emergency, you can make a 5 percent solution of simple sugar syrup from white corn syrup. Mix one part syrup with 19 parts plain tap water. A full measuring teaspoon contains about 0.2 ounces (5 ml) of liquid; an ordinary measuring cup contains approximately 8 ounces (250 ml). One teaspoon of white corn syrup mixed into approximately

three-quarters of a cup of water produces a solution that is just a little greater than 5 percent. Do not make the solution stronger than 5 percent. A more concentrated solution will not provide the correct fluid balance for the kittens.

A failing 4-ounce (100-g) kitten needs to receive about a teaspoonful (5 ml) of this simple sugar solution immediately. It should receive another teaspoonful in 30 minutes, and a teaspoonful at hourly intervals for three or four hours. After a few hours, the kitten should receive a mixture of one-half milk replacement formula and one-half simple sugar solution for two feedings. It should then receive the milk formula as detailed in Chapter 5.

You must give the homemade simple sugar solution to your kittens by mouth. This type of solution is not sterile. You must not administer it subcutaneously even if you have the equipment and know-how to do the procedure. Failing kittens will be too weak to suck from a bottle. The ideal method of feeding the solution to them is with a stomach tube. Unfortunately, stomach tubes may not be available in emergencies. If you absolutely must use an eyedropper, remember that these weak kittens can easily get fluid into their lungs. If they do, they will probably not survive. Chapters 6 and 7 explain feeding methods and equipment.

Your kittens have a better chance to survive if you use professional solutions and equipment than if you rely on makeshifts.

Human infants who need fluid therapy often receive a prescription liquid that contains water, dextrose (a simple sugar), and salt. If you can obtain this liquid, use it for your kittens. If you cannot, do not try to add table salt to your homemade fluid. Calculating the correct amount of salt is too difficult; too much salt can be very harmful.

Chapter Three

Housing and Caring for Orphaned Kittens

A pregnant cat selects a secluded, enclosed place in which to bear her litter. After her kittens are born, she keeps them warm with heat from her body. Kittens' natural instinct is to seek warmth and crawl toward their mother's body. Kittens have a very strong sucking reflex that will prompt them to seek a nipple and to fill their tiny stomachs with milk. The mother cat licks the kittens as they nurse, stimulating them to eliminate and removing their waste material to keep the nest clean.

When you raise orphaned kittens, you must perform all the tasks of the mother cat. Chapters 5, 6, and 7 detail the feeding of your orphans. However, food is not kittens' only necessity. If you want your orphaned kittens to thrive, you have to keep them safe. You have to keep them warm. You have to keep them clean.

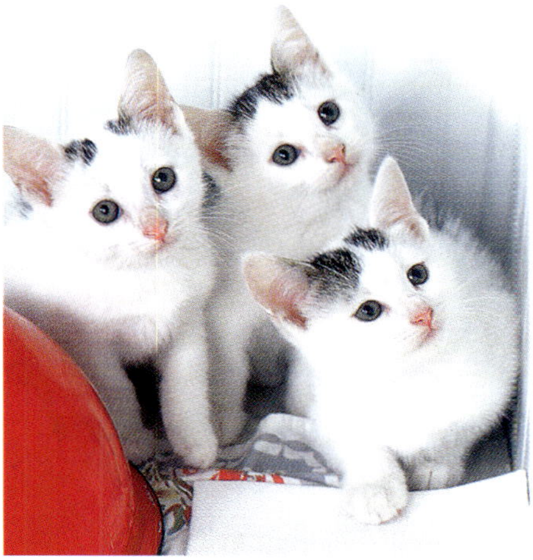

These three kittens are growing up healthy. As newborns, they were housed separately.

House Each Kitten Alone

Never house all your newborn kittens together in one box. Every normal baby mammal, including every kitten, is born with a very strong sucking reflex. In the absence of a mother cat's mammary glands upon which to suckle, nursing kittens will suck on any available structure of similar size, even though this sucking act does not provide nourishment. Motherless kittens (and most other young mammals) will suck on each other and cause serious damage to the ears and genitals of their littermates.

Your kittens will suck on each other even if you feed them an adequate volume of formula. If a mother cat were present to feed the kittens, each would nurse for only a few minutes at a time. However, each would nurse up to 30 times in a 24-hour period. You will be feeding your orphans only four to six times in the same 24 hours. You will give each kitten a much larger volume of formula at each feeding than it would consume if it were able to nurse from its mother whenever it wished to do so. However, even if you could offer all of the kittens a bottle every hour of every day and night, they would still suck on each other because they are born with a strong instinct to nurse.

Keeping each kitten in its own little bed has another advantage. Keeping each of them clean is easier. If any develop abnormal stools, you will be able to tell which ones they are. The disadvantage of keeping kittens apart is that this requires more space and equipment than housing the kittens together.

Making a Bed

A cardboard box is a satisfactory enclosure for each of your kittens. Cardboard beer cartons are good to use for this purpose because they are sturdy and convenient in size. Different brands vary, but a beer carton is approximately 11 or 12 inches wide, 16 inches long, and 8 inches deep (30 cm wide, 40 cm long, and 20 cm deep). The nearest adult beverage store can supply you with several of these cartons—try to get extras so you can replace any that become soiled or damaged. If you explain that you need them for newborn kittens, most proprietors will be sympathetic and will save cartons for you. If beer cartons are in short supply, any boxes of similar size (and most adult beverages are shipped to liquor stores in cartons) will serve the purpose.

Until the kittens are two or three weeks of age, each kitten does not need an entire carton for itself. You can divide one carton in half to make beds for two kittens. Keeping each tiny kitten in a half carton is more convenient. Supplying the necessary bedding and heat to the smaller space is easier and less costly.

Make a divider out of a separate piece of cardboard by notching both the carton and the cardboard halfway down and fitting the notches together. A bread knife or an electric carving knife is an excellent tool with which to make the notches.

When your kittens reach two and a half to three weeks of age, they will no longer require artificial heat. You can pull out the divider and use the whole box for just one kitten. Repair weakened boxes with duct tape.

A 10-by-16-inch (25-by-40-cm) box is enough space for a single kitten from three weeks of age until it is weaned to solid food. However, the box may not be deep enough. If a kitten can reach the top of the box with its paws, it will be able to climb

When your kittens are about four or five weeks of age and are eating well by themselves, you can put them back together in a larger, deeper box or cage. Until they no longer have the tendency to suck on each other, you must house them separately.

out. You might have to provide deeper boxes once your kittens are three weeks old.

Place your newborn kittens' beds into a warm, draft-free location near an electric outlet. You will need the outlet, or several outlets, to plug in the heating pad(s) to keep the kittens warm. Be careful about overloading circuits if you need to use several heating pads. If you blow the fuses, not only will you be in the dark but your kittens might become chilled before you discover the outage.

If your cardboard cartons come with attached lids, cut them off with a serrated knife like a bread knife. Do not close the lids of the boxes. Closed boxes easily overheat. If your room is not warm, cover part of each box with thin cloth such as a piece of an old sheet. To be sure that the covering cannot fall into the box on top of the kitten, attach the cloth to the box with spring clothespins.

Proper Bedding

You should use a type of bedding that will enable you to keep the kittens clean, dry, and uninjured. Bedding for your kittens must be soft since rough surfaces will cause newborn kittens to scrape their navel areas as they crawl. Bedding must be absorbent to soak up urine. Bedding must be easy and inexpensive to change.

Newspapers are absolutely unsatisfactory bedding for your kittens. They are neither soft nor absorbent, although they are inexpensive. Terry cloth towels are not much better. They have loops in which the kittens will catch their claws and possibly injure their paws. The best bedding for kittens is human babies' cloth diapers that are laundered and reused. Unfortunately, the disposable paper diapers for children are all made with elastic leg openings, so you cannot lay them flat to line a box.

Several layers of soft, high-quality paper towels can be used as disposable bedding for kittens. These can be placed over terry cloth towels in the bottom of each box. Unfortunately, inexpensive paper towels are usually too rough to be satisfactory. Disposable paper shop towels used as hand wipes by mechanics are even better than rolls of paper towels from the grocery store. Some of these can be laundered and reused several times before they fall apart.

You can cut into pieces any kind of absorbent, nonloopy cloth and use this for kittens' bedding. You can make good bedding by cutting old cotton baby blankets or flannel sheets into the right-sized pieces. Neighborhood garage sales are excellent sources for this kind of

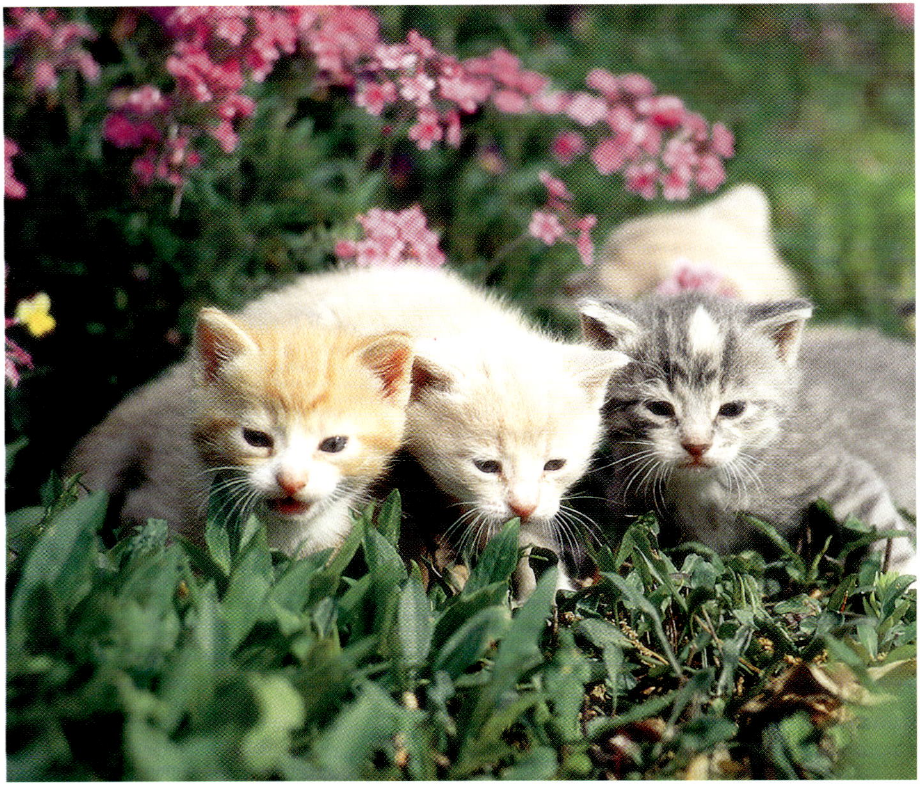

These kittens are old enough to withstand the great outdoors.

material. Boxes can be lined with pieces cut from a woven paper product designed to cover doctors' examining tables.

Even with appropriate bedding, the kittens may snag their nails on the material. If this is a problem, use a regular human fingernail trimmer to clip off only the tips of the tiny nails. You usually need to trim only the front claws.

Whatever bedding you choose, obtain a large supply. Even though you will stimulate your kittens to urinate and defecate after each feeding, the bedding will become wet or soiled at times. Have enough spare bedding on hand to change each box three or four times a day—several rolls of paper towels or several pieces of cloth, depending on how often you launder them. If you use cloth diapers, you might want to cut them in half and line each side of a divided carton individually. One cloth diaper is big enough to line both sides of a divided carton. If you use one whole, uncut diaper for two kittens and only one soils its bed, you will have to change both beds.

Keeping Newborns Warm

At birth, kittens have little ability to regulate their own body temperatures. Chilling is very harmful to newborn kittens. Severe or prolonged chilling often results in permanent damage to the kittens.

During the first few hours after the birth of a normal litter, the queen does not leave her kittens. She stays with her newborns, keeping them warm and fed. When the kittens are 24 hours old, the queen will leave them only long enough for her to eat and eliminate. While she is gone, the kittens huddle together and keep each other warm. When you hand-raise a litter, the mother is not present, and the kittens are housed separately. You must therefore supply the warmth necessary to keep your kittens healthy.

Newborn kittens develop the ability to regulate their body temperatures over a period of many days. Until the age of three weeks, kittens need a constant supply of artificial heat close to the normal body temperature of their mother. This is approximately 102°F (38.9°C). After three to four weeks, kittens can do well at a normal room temperature of 75°F (23.9°C). They will need artificial heat for a longer time if you keep them in a cold room.

Always be sure that your kittens cannot contact the heating pad directly. They could be severely burned.

The best way to supply this warmth is by using an ordinary commercial electric heating pad, available at every drug store. The pad must be placed underneath a kitten's box, *never* inside the box. If the pad is inside the box with a kitten, the kitten could crawl under the bedding and be burned or overheated by direct contact with the pad.

The heating pad should not extend under the entire box. Each of the kittens' areas should have a warm side and a cool side so that the kitten can crawl to whichever area is most comfortable for it. Commercial heating pads vary in size, but most are approximately 12 inches wide by 15 inches long (30 cm by 38 cm). When properly placed between two boxes, one pad can warm four enclosures for four separate kittens.

Heat lamps and even lightbulbs have been used to keep kittens warm. These are much less successful than electric heating pads. You always run the danger of a kitten becoming burned, dehydrated, or overheated from a bulb.

You should arrange the enclosures for newborn kittens so that the heat on the surface of the bedding where the kittens lie is maintained at 95 to 100°F (35 to 37.7°C). Temperatures as high as 104°F (40°C) are not harmful as long as the kittens have the opportunity to crawl to a cooler portion of their boxes. If the bedding is below 90°F (32.2°C), newborn kittens may become chilled. Kittens need artificial heat until they are at least three weeks of age.

Check the temperature of the bedding by placing a thermometer next to the kitten. Allow the thermometer sufficient time (ten minutes) to register before you read the temperature. An ordinary room thermometer will do the job. With a little practice, you can learn to tell if the bedding is near the correct temperature by feeling the surface. Since a human's body temperature is about 98.6°F (37°C), bedding at 100°F (37.7°C) feels warm to the touch but does not feel hot.

Commercial electric heating pads usually have three control settings: high, medium, and low. These settings are not sufficiently accurate to regulate a kitten's heat supply. Experiment a little to adjust the heat to 100°F (37.7°C) at the surface of the bedding. Place the bedding into the box. Place the thermometer onto the bedding. Arrange the heating pad underneath the box, and turn it on low. If the temperature reaches 100°F (37.7°C) in ten minutes, you have found the correct setting.

In many instances, the temperature will be below 100°F (37.7°C) at the low setting. If this happens, try the medium setting. Often, electric pads will deliver too much heat at medium. To reduce the temperature to approximately 100°F (37.7°C), place a folded towel between the heating pad and the box. Determine the necessary thickness of the towel by checking the thermometer. If the bedding is too warm, add another fold of towel. If too cold, remove one. Almost no electric heating pad will need to be adjusted to high to deliver 100°F (37.7°C) of heat to the bedding through the bottom of the box.

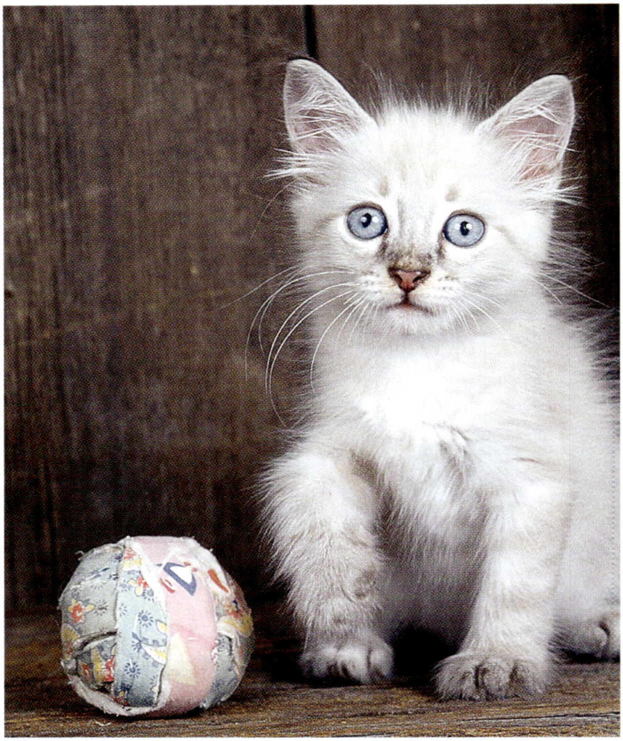

Raised by hand—a healthy and happy kitten!

Check the temperature for each box and each heating pad. Never trust the heating pads to deliver the same temperatures even if they are identical. Recheck the temperature in each box daily for the first few days and occasionally thereafter. Correct temperatures are too essential during the first few days of kittens' lives to take chances.

When your baby kittens are between three and four weeks of age, you can turn off the heating pad during the day if you have a warm room (75°F [23.9°C]) in which to

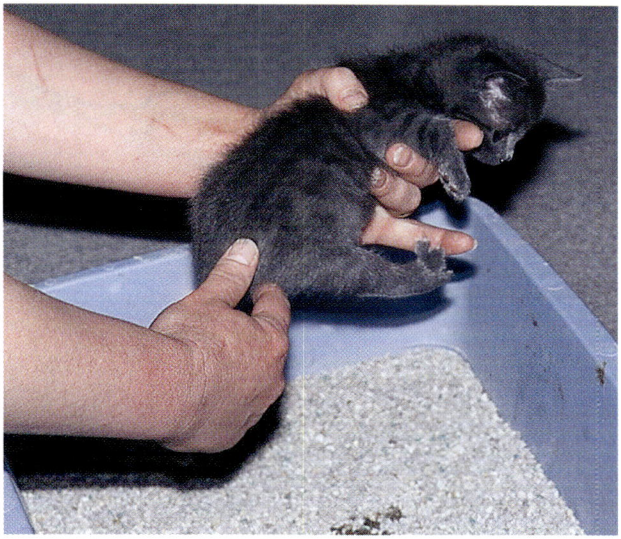

This kitten is being stimulated to eliminate.

keep the kittens. Turn the pad on again if the room gets cool at night. At four weeks of age, your kittens will be fine in any room where most people feel comfortable without wearing a sweater.

Keeping Kittens Clean

A normal mother cat produces all the food and warmth her kittens need. She also keeps them clean. She licks their anal and genital areas while they nurse, which stimulates them to urinate and defecate. She ingests the kittens' waste material, thereby keeping their nest area free of waste material.

This sounds disgusting, but nature has its own way of solving problems that would otherwise become serious. Suppose a mother cat did not ingest her kittens' waste—what would the nest be like in a few days?

When you hand-raise kittens, you have two choices. No, licking is not one of them. First, you can clean up messes on the bedding. Second, you can stimulate each kitten to urinate and defecate after you feed it and then wipe away its eliminations. If you do not stimulate the kittens to eliminate and then clean them up, they will mess later and you will have to change their bedding very often. If you do stimulate them, the kittens will not usually eliminate again until the next time they are fed, so they will keep their beds clean.

Here is how to stimulate a kitten to eliminate. Use a cotton ball. Moisten it with warm water. *Gently* stroke the anal and genital areas of each kitten as soon as you have fed it. In most cases, each kitten will urinate and defecate in response to this stimulus. Then all you have to do is to wipe away the waste and return the kitten to its clean bed.

If the kitten does not eliminate in response to *gentle* stimulation, put it back into its bed. Try again to stimulate it to eliminate after you have fed its littermates. If it still does not defecate and urinate, do not continue to rub the kitten until you have irritated its anal area. Put it back into its bed, and try again later. Change its bedding if you find that it is dirty or wet.

Evidence shows that kittens under 14 days of age cannot eliminate spontaneously. Unless their mother licks them to stimulate urination and

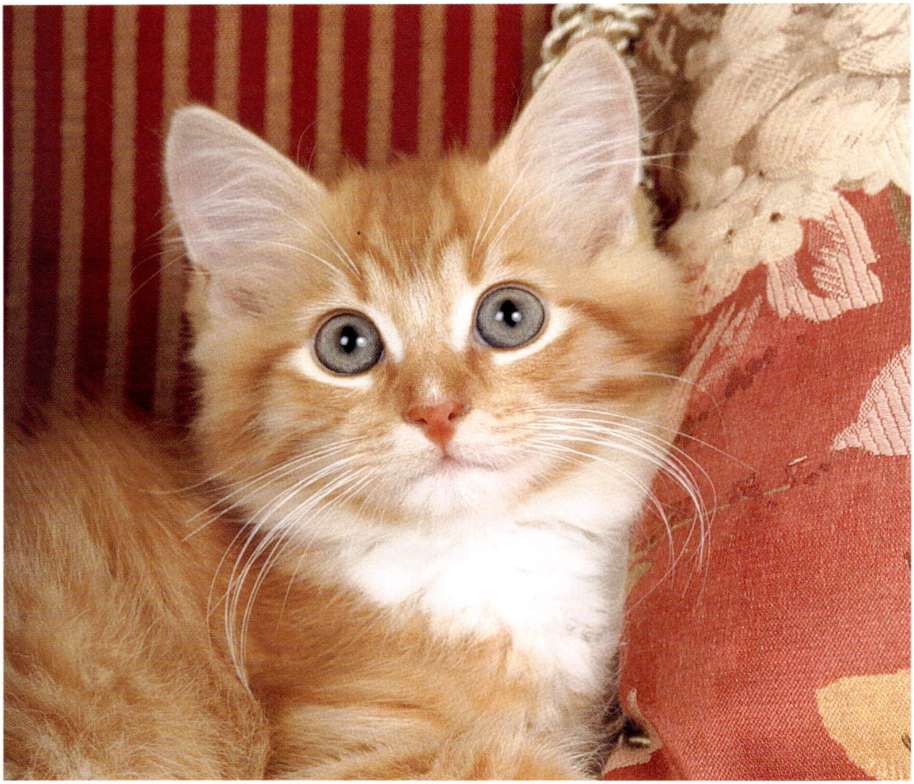

With the proper care and housing, your hand-raised kitten will grow up strong.

defecation, they may die of intestinal stasis and absorbed toxins. Veterinarians do not know if this is true of every kitten, but do not take chances. While your kittens are less than two weeks old, stimulate them to eliminate at least three times a day.

With your litter of orphaned kittens snug in individual warm, soft, clean compartments, you are well on your way to providing everything they need to thrive. All that remains is to provide the kittens with an appropriate diet and a way for them to consume it. The next three chapters will show you how to select the correct food and how to get the kittens to consume it.

Chapter Four

Feline Nutrition from Birth to Weaning

Mother Nature always knows best. Mother's milk provides optimum nutrition for the newborn animal. Nature changes the composition of mother's milk to suit the needs of the growing young. A person who undertakes the hand-raising of orphaned mammals has taken on a formidable task. That person must provide nutrition that is as near as possible to the animals' mother's milk.

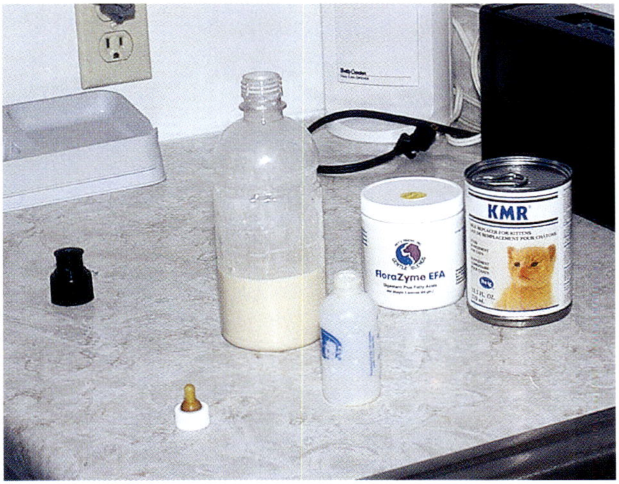

Assemble everything you will need to feed the kittens.

Composition of Queens' Colostrum and Milk

The milk produced by a mother animal immediately after giving birth to her young is *colostrum*. The composition of colostrum gradually changes to the composition of the mother's normal milk over a few days. Colostrum differs from mature milk in several important ways.

- Colostrum contains many proteins that enhance kittens' resistance to disease organisms.
- Colostrum is generally lower in protein, fat, and lactose than the milk produced later.
- Colostrum is lower in total solids and therefore higher in moisture than mature milk.

These facts are important to people hand-raising orphaned kittens from birth. Kittens are much more likely to do well if they have had colostrum from their mothers. No other milk can duplicate the immunoglobulins (antibodies) found

only in colostrum and that the kittens' intestines absorb for only the first few hours after birth. Kittens that have not received colostrum need special attention to prevent them from contracting disease.

The intestines of newborn animals are not yet completely developed. Oversupply of some nutrients to very young animals causes diarrhea, dehydration, and death. Undernourished baby animals are vastly more likely to survive than are overnourished babies. Kittens' intestines at birth are able to handle colostrum but are not able to absorb the milk their mothers will produce later.

Mature milk is composed of water, fat, protein, and lactose. The tiny fraction called *ash* is made of minerals and other substances.

Lactose, or milk sugar, is a disaccharide composed of two molecules of simple sugars. As a complex molecule, the lactose must be digested by the kitten before the body can use it for energy.

No artificial milk can be formulated that exactly duplicates the milk of a normal mother cat. The table illustrates the different compositions of mother's milk of some common species.

The values in the table come from information recently published by W. L. Hurley, Ph.D. Dr. Hurley is a leading lactation biologist from the University of Illinois. Some references give different percentages of protein, fat, and total solids, which are usually lower than those in the table. Why do the values differ?

- The composition of humans' and cows' milk has been determined by analyzing thousands of samples. It is likely that some of the values listed for the composition of the milk of dogs and cats have been determined from only a few samples.
- It is known that the composition of milk of every nursing mother changes as her infants grow. The variation in values for dogs' and cats' milk may have been determined at different stages of lactation.
- Just as with milk from different breeds of cows, there may be significant differences between the milk of various breeds of cats and dogs.

The Composition of Milk of Different Species

(Approximate % of each component, values calculated to nearest ½%)

Species	*Protein*	*Fat*	*Lactose*	*Total Solids*	*Moisture*
Cat	11%	11%	3.5%	25%	75%
Dog	9.5%	8%	3.5%	20%	80%
Cow	3%	3.5%	5%	12%	88%
Human	1%	4.5%	7%	13%	87%

Commercial Milk Replacements

Whole 3.5 percent cows' milk is not adequate for kittens. Ordinary homogenized milk purchased at grocery stores is standardized to contain 3.5 percent butterfat by weight. The dairy industry calls this product *whole milk.*

- The percentages of both protein and fat in cats' milk are more than triple the percentages of these substances in 3.5 percent cows' milk.
- The percentage of total solids in cats' milk is double that in cows' milk.

Obviously, ordinary 3.5 percent cows' milk is not an adequate diet on which to raise orphaned kittens. What can you use that is more nutritionally correct?

Commercial Products for Orphaned Kittens

Several feline milk replacements are available in pet and feed stores. Nutritionists scientifically formulate commercial milk replacements to replace queens' milk. These preparations are sold in liquid and powdered forms. When *moisture* is listed as an ingredient of a commercially prepared food, the moisture is water. The words *total solids* or *dry matter* in an ingredients list mean everything in the product except water.

Using these products is the most convenient and satisfactory way to feed orphaned kittens. Commercial milk replacements have only a few disadvantages:

1. Commercial feline milk replacements may be difficult to obtain in some localities.

2. These products appear to be expensive to use. However, compared with the cost of the ingredients needed to produce satisfactory home-formulated replacements, the commercial products may actually be less expensive than formulas you make yourself.

3. If you have only one or two kittens to feed, even the small 5-ounce (150-ml) cans of the ready-to-use milk may spoil before the kittens consume it all. You can instead prepare the powdered product in small quantities as needed.

4. Some of the products sold in powdered form are difficult to prepare. Simply stirring the powder into water may result in a mixture that is too lumpy to pass through the hole of a nipple. To prepare these products more easily, try the following tips:

- Always add the powder to the water, not the water to the powder.
- Sprinkle the powder into the water a little at a time. Mix well before each addition of powder.
- Use cold water to mix the formula, and warm the mixture just before feeding.
- Mix the formula with a blender if you have one. If not, use a wire wisk or a fork.

Commercial substitutes for queens' milk are formulated to contain from 7 to 8 percent protein, 4 to

5 percent fat, and 80 to 82 percent moisture. If you examine the packages of the powdered commercial products, you will see values such as: protein, 40 percent; fat, 25 percent; moisture, 5 percent. These determinations are made on a dry basis. When you add the correct amount of water to the products, the protein, fat, and moisture values approximate those in the liquids.

The values of nutrients in the commercial products do not equal the values given in the table for queens' milk. Most likely, the manufacturers of these products used values calculated by different researchers. Whichever values are actually the most accurate does not matter. Kittens will live and grow to weaning when fed commercial formulas.

Dilute the Formula for Newborns

If your kittens have just been born, you must adjust their formula to resemble that of their mother's colostrum. You cannot add the immunoglobulins found in natural colostrum, but you can approximate a milk formula that your kittens can digest.

Even if you feed commercial canned kitten formula, add one-third the volume in extra water for the first two days. Yes, your kittens will receive fewer nutrients in the diluted formula. Their intestines are not well-enough developed to handle those additional nutrients, but the kittens need the extra water to keep their bodies hydrated.

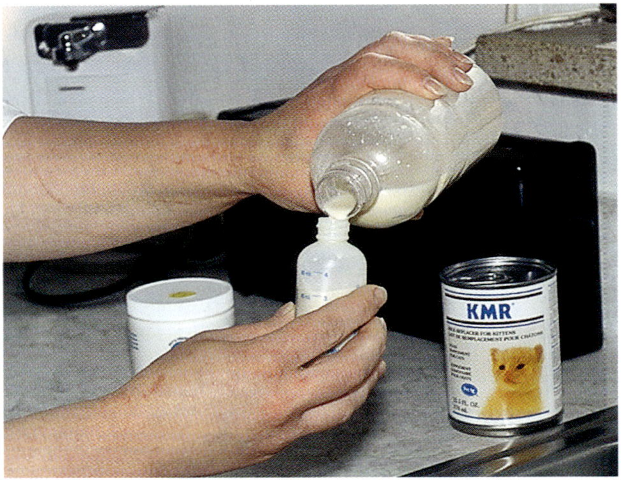

For the third, fourth, and fifth days of life, add only one-fourth volume (not one-third) of extra water to the kittens' formula. On the sixth day, use the formula without diluting it additionally with water. Observe your kittens' stools at least three times a day. If the stools are not formed, dilute the formula with one-third more water until the kittens pass soft, yellowish, but formed stools.

Be sure to measure accurately and keep everything clean.

Homemade Milk Substitutes

Homogenized cows' milk alone is an inadequate substitute for queens' milk. You can add various substances to ordinary 3.5 percent

Important!
Dilute newborn kittens' formula with one-third volume (30 percent) extra water.

Homemade Formulas for Orphaned Kittens

Product	*Additives*
Commercial liquid or dry products	Mix and feed as directed on the package
⅔ cup 3.5% milk	⅓ cup nonfat dry milk and 1 tablespoon vegetable oil
⅔ cup 3.5% milk	½ cup 18% coffee cream
1 cup 3.5% milk	¼ cup 30% whipping cream
1 cup evaporated whole milk	½ cup water

homogenized milk to improve its nutritional value for kittens.

Using 3.5 Percent Milk

Nonfat dry milk is milk from which most of the moisture and all of the fat have been removed. It is sold as a powder that mixes easily with water. Nonfat dry milk can be used to increase the protein and total solids in cows' milk. Mixing instructions are printed on each box of nonfat dry milk. Most brands indicate using one-third volume of the product mixed with three volumes of water to prepare the equivalent of liquid nonfat milk.

If you mix one-third cup of nonfat dry milk powder with two-thirds cup of whole 3.5 percent milk instead of water, the percentage of protein doubles (from 3 percent to 6 percent). The percentage of total solids also doubles (from 12 percent to 24 percent) in the mixed liquid. This formula will be deficient in fat for your kittens. It will contain only the fat contained in the two-thirds cup of whole milk, which is far less fat than the kittens require. To increase the percentage of fat, mix one tablespoon of vegetable oil into a cup of the mixture. Be sure to mix well before each feeding.

Coffee cream sold in grocery stores in one-half pint or pint cartons contains 18 percent butterfat. If you mix one part of 18 percent cream with two parts 3.5 percent milk, the resulting liquid contains about 8 percent butterfat. This amount is satisfactory to feed to kittens over a week of age. Regular *whipping cream* contains 30 percent butterfat. If you mix your kittens' formula with 30 percent cream, use one part cream to four parts regular 3.5 percent milk. This mixture con-

tains nearly 9 percent butterfat. *Heavy whipping cream* contains 40 percent butterfat. If you use 40 percent cream, dilute one part cream with six parts regular 3.5 percent milk to make a formula containing approximately 9 percent butterfat. Remember to dilute all formulas for newborns. This approximates the analysis of their mothers' colostrum.

Using Human Infant Formulas

Examine the values of protein, fat, and total solids of the milk of different species. Cats' milk is much higher in each of these ingredients than is humans' milk. Using a canned product manufactured for human babies is not likely to be satisfactory for raising orphaned kittens. Human infant formulas are not less expensive than products made especially for kittens. For these reasons, do not use canned or powdered milk products designed for human infants to feed orphaned kittens.

Evaporated milk is 3.5 percent cows' milk from which one-half of the water has been removed before the milk is processed. Some brands of evaporated milk contain added calcium and/or vitamin D. Evaporated milk is designed to provide a more creamlike product to use in cooking, baking, or beverages. Evaporated milk is not the same as *condensed milk,* which contains added sugar. Evaporated milk is also not the same as *evaporated skimmed milk* or *lite evaporated milk,* which has had the fat removed.

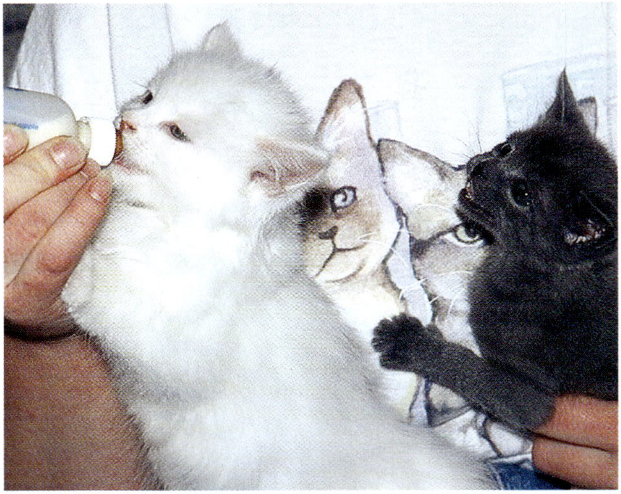

Growing kittens require a lot of milk.

Do not feed either condensed milk or lite milk to kittens.

Evaporated milk straight from the can (undiluted) contains about 24 percent solids and 76 percent water. If you dilute evaporated milk with an equal volume of water, you will prepare milk containing the nutritional equivalent of whole 3.5 percent milk. If you dilute canned evaporated milk with only one-half an equal volume of water, your preparation will contain 18 percent solids and 82 percent water. Diluting evaporated milk this way makes a fairly satisfactory substitute for commercial kitten milk once your kittens are about a week old.

Many pet books recommend a formula for kittens and puppies consisting of various amounts, usually 8 ounces (250 ml), of homogenized milk with the addition of one or two raw egg yolks. This mixture can be prepared to be nutritionally

adequate. However, the feeding of uncooked eggs cannot be recommended. Even raw eggs in the shell have been found to contain *Salmonella* bacteria. Uncooked or undercooked eggs have been implicated in food poisoning of both humans and animals.

If you do use raw eggs to feed kittens, mix the formula fresh for each feeding. Do not keep any unused formula (even refrigerated) for more than eight hours. Do not ever warm a milk formula containing raw egg more than once. You can make better, safer, and cheaper homemade formulas for feeding orphaned kittens than those containing raw eggs.

Homemade Diet Tips

Remember, for newborn kittens, add one-third to one-fourth more moisture to each of the formulas to approximate the values of colostrum. This is so important that it cannot be repeated too often.

Consider replacing your homemade formulas with commercial kittens' milk as soon as you can. Your kittens will probably grow faster and remain in better condition when fed a diet formulated for the purpose than when fed a homemade diet.

Stir or shake each preparation before every feeding to assure that the ingredients are well mixed. Store milk formula in the refrigerator. Do not pour unconsumed warmed milk back into the refrigerated container. Unused warmed milk may be contaminated; discard it.

Buying milk additives such as cream and powdered nonfat milk for your kittens is less satisfactory and not less expensive than buying milk formulated especially for kittens. If economy is a consideration, buy the powdered kitten product, and mix it yourself. If convenience is more important, buy the canned kitten milk.

Nature is very forgiving. That is why kittens survive on a great variety of homemade formulas. Even if your milk formula is less than ideal, you can keep kittens alive until they are old enough to eat solid food. The kittens' growth rate will be slower if their diet is deficient in nutrients and total solids. However, they will catch up when they are weaned and are eating a good quality kitten food.

A Practical Feeding Schedule for Orphaned Kittens

7:00 A.M.
1:00 P.M.
7:00 P.M.
MIDNIGHT

Feeding Schedule

Kittens nursing from their mothers will suckle 10 to 20 times a day, taking only a little milk each time. Wild species of felines nurse their kittens

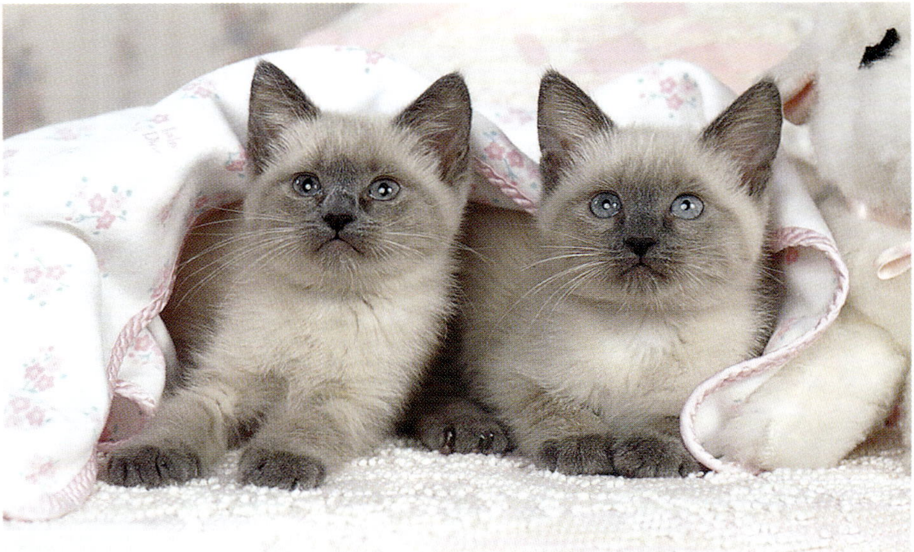

Whether purebreds or mixed breeds, all can be raised to be healthy pets.

much less frequently since the wild mother must spend a significant amount of time away from her litter while she hunts for food.

A person hand-raising a litter of orphaned kittens will find that feeding them every two hours is neither practical nor necessary. Unless the kittens are very weak, a feeding every six hours will allow them to get enough nourishment to live and grow until they are weaned. Even a feeding every eight hours will be sufficient to keep kittens alive until weaning.

If more than one person can feed the orphans, you can adjust the schedule.

Kittens do not do well if fed less than every eight hours. If you have a full-time job that requires you to spend more than eight hours away from home, ask your boss if you can take your kittens to work with you. You will be surprised at how many bosses will be sympathetic to the kittens' plight.

Proper Feeding Amounts

The way you feed the kittens affects the amount they ingest. The following discusses food amounts when bottle-feeding and when tube-feeding.

Bottle-feeding

If you bottle-feed orphaned kittens and they have normal formed stools, feed as much as the kittens will take at each feeding. If a kitten does not take about 0.1 ounces (3 or 4 ml) for every 4 ounces (100 g) of its body weight, check the temperature of the

Each kitten consumes a whole bottle full of formula.

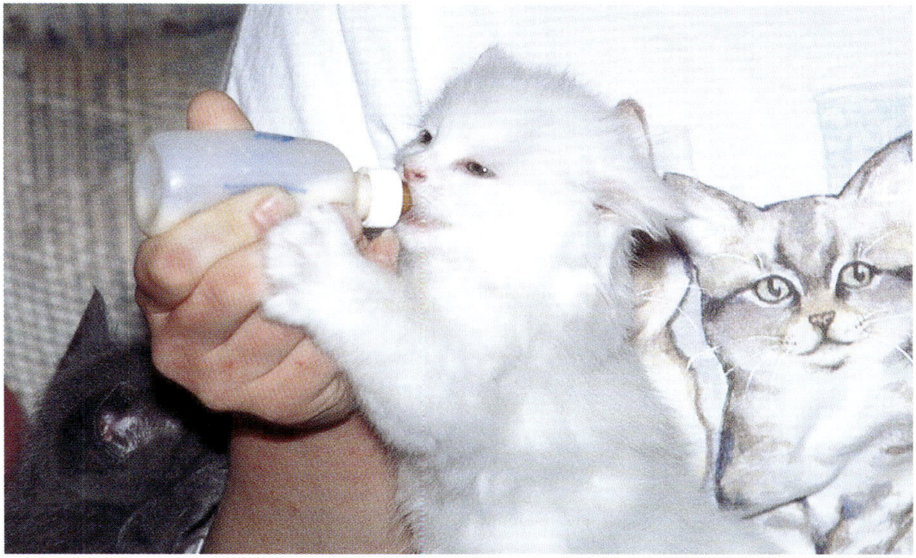

formula. Give the kitten another turn at the bottle after the others have been fed.

Tube-Feeding

Before you attempt to use a stomach tube (feeding tube) to feed your kittens, read Chapter 6. That chapter contains detailed instructions about using the necessary equipment.

Tube-fed kittens have no choice; they receive the amount you put into their stomachs. Tube-fed kittens should receive 0.3 ounces (8 to 10 ml) of formula for every 4 ounces (100 g) of their body weight. Divide this amount into three or four daily feedings. A newborn 4-ounce (100-g) kitten should receive about 0.1 ounces (3 ml) of formula every six hours.

If you give a kitten too much milk by tube, the excess will run out of its mouth. This is potentially harmful. The overfed kitten may breathe the milk into its lungs and develop aspiration pneumonia. Give the formula slowly at first. At the first sign of milk appearing in a kitten's mouth, *stop!* Check to be sure that the tube has not been partially withdrawn. If it has, replace the tube. If the tube is still in place, give the kitten less formula the next time.

Normal Growth Rate

When raised by the mother, kittens usually double their birth weight during their first week of life. They often gain 4 ounces (100 g) a week until weaning. Kittens in small litters with well-nourished mothers

will grow faster than those in litters of five or more or with mothers who eat limited amounts of nutritious food.

Hand-raised kittens are likely to grow at a slower rate. Kittens' mothers can do a much better job of raising their young than can the best-intentioned person.

Failure to grow is a danger sign in hand-raised kittens. If your kittens do not increase in weight by 1 ounce (30 g) during the first week and nearly 2 ounces (50 g) a week thereafter, something is wrong.

- Observe the kittens' stools. These should be formed but not hard. Liquid stools indicate a problem with infection, parasites, or an indigestible formula.
- Feed the kittens more often. Bottle-fed kittens that do not grow may be unable to consume the volume of formula they need.
- Feed tube-fed kittens more at each feeding. Perhaps you did not calculate the correct amount to feed them.
- Check your formula. If your kittens' stools are normal but the kittens fail to gain weight, perhaps you need to alter the formula.

Weigh Your Kittens Often

Check your kittens' weight gain at least every three days. A very useful type of scale for this purpose is one made for weighing food portions. These scales are relatively inexpensive, durable, and calibrated in both ounces and grams. Food scales can usually weigh amounts up to 10 pounds (4.5 kg), although your kittens will be too big and active to sit in the food basket by the time they weigh about 2 pounds (1 kg).

You can use a postal scale until your kittens weigh more than 1 pound (0.5 kg). Place each kitten into a light box, weigh the kitten and the box, weigh the box alone, then subtract the weight of the box. Some scales can be adjusted to register zero with the box in place. Ordinary bathroom scales are not sufficiently sensitive to weigh an animal of less than 10 pounds (4.5 kg).

Keep a pencil and paper handy near your scales. Each time you weigh the kittens, write it on the day's record page. Doing so will allow you to detect most problems before they become serious.

Chapter Five

Feeding Tools for Kittens

The best formulas in the world will not keep orphaned kittens alive if you cannot get the food into their stomachs. Mother cats never have a problem. Instinct causes their kittens to seek a nipple and to suck until their stomachs are filled. What factors promote this instinctive behavior?

1. The kittens' empty stomachs produce the feeling of hunger.

2. The mother's body heat attracts the kittens to her.

3. Her nipples provide a protruding structure upon which the kittens can suck.

4. The queen's milk has a distinct odor and taste that the kittens instinctively desire.

The first three factors cause kittens to suck on each other if they have no mother on which to nurse. The kittens are hungry, their littermates are warm, they can find paws or genitals that protrude and can be sucked. Kittens will damage each other by continuously sucking on body parts. This is why you should house them individually until they are able to consume solid food.

You must not only house the orphans appropriately and provide a correct milk formula for them, but you must also arrange for them to consume the formula at regular intervals. Only two devices will allow you to do this safely, consistently, and quickly.

Commercial Pet-Feeding Bottles

Bottles designed for human infants have been available for decades. Throughout the years, these bottles have undergone changes. The first bottles were simple glass containers with rubber nipples stretched over the top. Human nursing bottles and nipples are now available in a wide variety of configurations. These include breast-shaped nipples and bottles with collapsible plastic liners. The most common styles of human nursing bottles are made of plastic. These have a screw-on collar that holds a flanged rubber nipple in place. Nipples for human infants are supplied in a few sizes. Those for

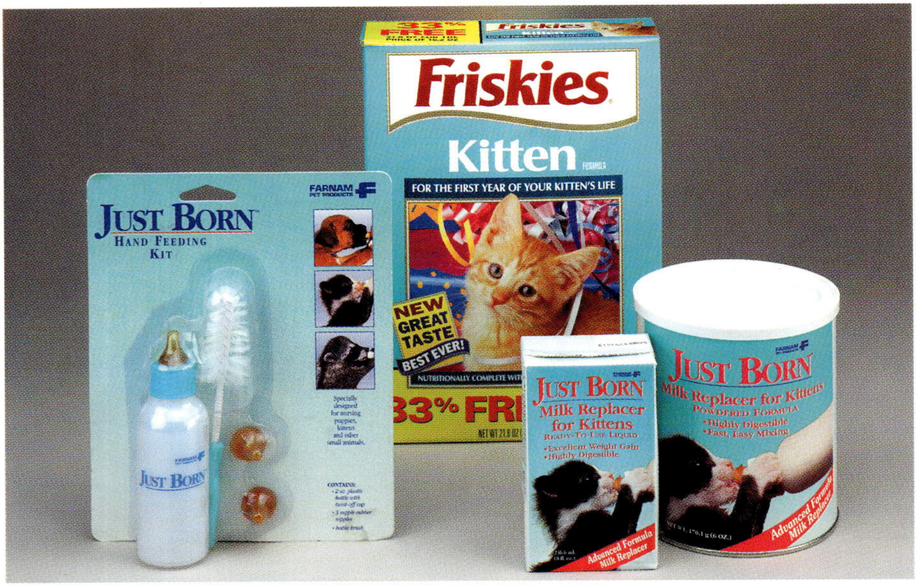

Many companies make suitable food for kittens.

premature or weak babies are made of softer material than those designed for babies capable of vigorous sucking.

The nipples provided by human baby bottles, even those for premature infants, are far too large to fit into a nursing kitten's mouth. Nipples intended for kittens and other tiny newborn animals are available in pet and feed stores.

Pick the Correct Nipple

Some manufacturers of pet nursing equipment have merely made copies of human bottles and nipples in various sizes, while other manufacturers have taken into consideration the way cat (and dog) anatomy differs from human anatomy. These manufacturers have designed their products with animal requirements in mind.

Differences in animal and human anatomy influence the correct shape of the nipple for each species.

1. The heads of cats and dogs are not the same shape as the heads of humans. Even kittens with relatively round heads have longer jaws than do humans. Kittens (and puppies) have longer noses, longer palates, and longer tongues.

2. The skin of a cat's mammary gland to which the nipple is attached is looser and more stretchable than the skin of a human's mammary gland. When it nurses, a kitten (or a puppy) draws the nipple farther into the back of its mouth than does a human infant.

Unlike human infants, kittens (and puppies) require relatively long, narrow nipples if they are to nurse properly. The presence of the nipple in

the back of the mouth stimulates the sucking reflex. When offered a nipple that is too short, kittens chew or mouth it in their attempts to get a good sucking grip. Eventually, kittens learn to suck the short nipple but never as actively as they can suck a longer one.

A commonly available pet-feeding set consists of a bottle and nipple that is a miniature replica of a human baby bottle. The entire nipple is less than ¾ inch (1.9 cm) long. The tip of the nipple is about ¼ inch (0.6 cm) wide by about ⅜ inch (1 cm) long. This nipple then abruptly enlarges to a diameter of about ½ inch (1.3 cm). Kittens cannot get the enlarged part of the nipples into their mouths. This means that the only part of the nipple on which a kitten can nurse is the ⅜-inch (1-cm) tip. Even newborn kittens prefer a longer nipple than this.

Some manufacturers supply kitten-feeding nipples that are longer, made of softer material, and taper more gradually. The nipples of one brand are more than an inch long. Although the tips of these nipples are also about ¼ inch (0.6 cm) in diameter, the sucking length is at least ⅝ inch (1.5 cm). Kittens can nurse from these nipples much more easily than they can nurse from the shorter ones.

If you can find them, buy the pet nursers with longer, softer, more conical nipples. If you cannot find them, try to make do with the short nipples until your local supplier can order better ones for your kittens.

Most nipples for pets are sold without holes in the tips. You must pierce them before kittens can draw out milk. Hold a small sewing needle with a pair of pliers; the needle will get too hot to hold with your bare fingers. Heat the needle in a flame or the burner of a stove. Touch the point of the hot needle to the tip of the nipple, pressing until it just pierces the rubber (or plastic) of the nipple. Withdraw the needle, fill a bottle with water, attach the pierced nipple, then test it for the correct flow.

Hold the bottle and nipple upside down. If the hole in the nipple is large enough for your kittens, water will drip out of the bottle in a slow flow of about two drops a second. If no water drips out, enlarge the hole in the nipple. Heat the needle again, and hold the hot needle in the hole just a moment longer to melt more of the rubber or plastic. Then test it again. Repeat until you get the hole just right.

If you accidentally get the hole in the nipple too large, a continuous stream of water will run out of the nipple when you hold the bottle upside down. If you made the hole too large, try boiling the nipple for a minute or two in a pan of water. Some nipples are made of a material that will swell up in boiling water. This makes the holes smaller.

Any bottle that you can attach the correct nipple to will adequately hold the kittens' formula. One brand of tiny little nipples is made to fit only on the manufacturer's tiny little bottles. Other brands of nipples will fit both the manufacturer's bottles and standard human baby bottles. Pet-feed-

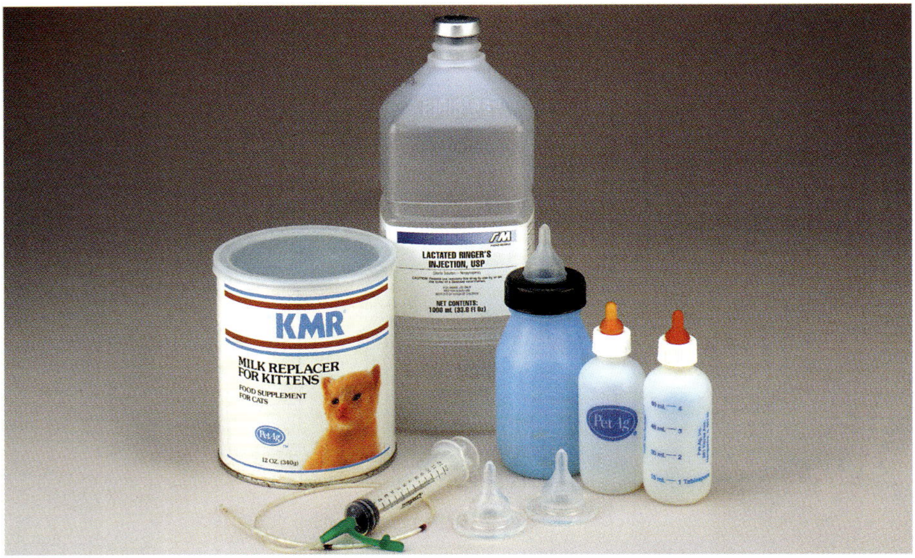

Bottles, nipples, stomach tubes, and hypodermic syringes are used to feed newborn kittens.

ing nipples are sold in packs of nipples only as well as in kits containing nipples, bottles, and bottle brushes for cleaning the little bottles. Human baby bottles are sold in every drugstore and are usually less expensive than those sold in pet shops for feeding animals. Brushes for cleaning standard baby bottles are displayed with the baby supplies in most drugstores. The standard 4-ounce (about 120-ml) size human baby bottles, either glass or plastic, are very satisfactory for feeding kittens.

Stomach Tubes and Hypodermic Syringes

An acceptable alternative method of feeding an orphaned newborn kitten is with a plastic tube inserted directly into its stomach. These tubes are called *nasogastric catheters.* They were originally designed for passing through a nostril and into the stomach of a human infant. When used for feeding a tiny newborn animal, do not pass the tube through the nostril. Pass a tube over the base of the tongue, down the esophagus, and into the stomach of the animal.

Stomach tubes are supplied in *french* sizes and in varying lengths. The appropriate tube with which to feed a newborn kitten is size 8 french, length 15 inches (38 cm). This tube is about ⅛ inch (0.3 cm) in diameter. It has a closed tip with two openings along the sides, ½ inch (1.3 cm) and ¼ inch (0.6 cm) from the end. The top of the tube is fitted with a plastic receptacle that fits onto a hypodermic syringe. A little plastic

capping device plugs the end of the tube to prevent liquid from flowing out when removing the tube from the syringe. This device serves no purpose in the feeding of kittens, and you can snip it off with a scissor to get it out of the way.

If the kittens are premature and very tiny, you may use a size 6 french feeding tube. The smaller the french number, the smaller the diameter of the tube. The smaller the diameter, the more easily you can pass the tube into the trachea instead of into the esophagus of the kitten. To minimize this problem, use the largest tube that can be passed without using any force. The tube should slip down the kitten's throat without resistance.

Milk is forced through the feeding tube and into the kitten's stomach by the use of a hypodermic syringe attached to the stomach tube. Hypodermic syringes are calibrated by the number of cubic centimeters (cc) they hold. One fluid ounce is 30 cc. Syringes are commonly supplied in 3 cc, 5 cc, and 12 cc sizes. Hypodermic syringes are made of plastic and are intended to be thrown away after each use, not sterilized and reused as were the old-fashioned glass syringes. However, plastic syringes will last through many cleanings and may be reused to feed kittens until the rubber end of the plunger disintegrates.

Even though you may not feed your newborns as much as 3 cc at a feeding, within a very few days they will require more than 3 cc each time you feed them. Obtain a syringe with which to start your kittens and several 12 cc syringes to use as they grow. If your syringes are supplied with aluminum hypodermic needles, remove the needles, and have your veterinarian dispose of them correctly. You have no use for the needles.

Obtain plastic stomach tubes and syringes from your veterinarian. Veterinarians buy the syringes by the hundreds for everyday use. They can order the nasogastric catheters (stomach tubes) from medical suppliers if they do not keep them on hand.

Eyedroppers—Emergency Use Only

Everyone has used an eyedropper for applying medication to their own eyes or noses, for measuring small amounts of liquids, even for adding food coloring to cake frosting. The eyedropper, glass or plastic, is a poor substitute for a bottle or a feeding tube as a piece of equipment with which to feed orphaned kittens.

- The kitten cannot suck on an eyedropper. It can only swallow the formula that you drop into its mouth.
- If you place more than a single drop (two drops at the most) of formula into a kitten's mouth at one time, the kitten is in danger of getting the milk down into its trachea and lungs instead of its esophagus and stomach. *Aspiration pneumonia*

commonly results from feeding a newborn kitten with a dropper.

- Using an eyedropper is extremely time consuming. The kitten must swallow every drop before you can introduce another drop into its mouth. If you try to feed even a few kittens with a dropper, plan on spending an hour at each feeding.

If you obtain newborn kittens in the middle of the night and have nothing else available with which to feed them, you can try to give the kittens a little nourishment with a dropper until the stores open in the morning. Then obtain better equipment. The only other valid excuse for feeding a newborn kitten with an eyedropper would be if you live in the middle of the desert and no stores are within a hundred miles.

If you ever use a dropper, be patient and careful. Never squirt too much milk into a kitten's mouth at one time. Be sure the milk does not enter a kitten's lungs. You might actually kill it with kindness.

Keeping Your Equipment Clean

A mother cat's skin and nipples are not sterile. Normal bacteria are present on her skin. However, the milk inside her glands is sterile, and the milk formula that you feed your kittens should be as bacteria-free as possible.

Warm milk formula is an excellent place for bacteria to grow. Never warm more milk than you will use at one feeding. Discard leftover formula, do not return it to the refrigerated container. The bacteria in warm milk may contaminate the whole supply.

After each use, wash everything that the milk formula touches—spoons, measuring cups, blenders, jars, bottles, nipples, syringes, and feeding tubes—thoroughly with hot soapy water. Use a bottle brush to scrub milk residue out of bottles; squirt hot suds many times through syringes and tubes. Rinse thoroughly with many changes of hot water. Store your equipment in a covered bowl to protect it between feedings.

You may feed an entire litter of healthy kittens with the same bottle and nipple, or tube and syringe, between cleaning the equipment. If any kitten appears not to be strong, particularly if it has watery diarrhea, feed it with its own equipment. If your kittens have any abnormal condition that bacteria or viruses may cause, sterilize all the equipment by boiling for 20 minutes in a pan of water. Do not take chances of spreading disease through contaminated bottles or tubes.

Chapter Six

How to Use the Tools to Feed Your Kittens

The pet-nursing bottle will be the main tool with which you will raise your orphans. Most people expect kittens to grab the nipple the first time they are offered it and to suck as much as their stomachs will hold. Every newborn, kitten and human alike, must learn to nurse from its mother or from nursing bottles.

Nature does a good job of teaching newborns to nurse from their mothers. Imitate nature as closely as you can. Normal, healthy kittens will learn to feed from the bottle within a few minutes.

What Can Go Wrong

When you feed kittens by hand, four things can go wrong:

1. *Underfeeding.* If you feed your kittens too little, they will be malnourished. If they receive nothing or nearly nothing, the kittens will starve.

2. *Overfeeding.* If you feed your kittens too much, they will have diarrhea, dehydration, and digestive problems. In severe cases, the kittens may die.

3. *Feeding the Wrong Formula.* Even if your formula is not exactly like their mothers' milk, most kittens will stay alive until they are able to eat solid food. The wrong formula may cause kittens to grow poorly and to have diarrhea.

4. *Aspiration Pneumonia.* This medical term means an inflammation of the lungs (pneumonia) caused by liquid being sucked into the trachea instead of the esophagus.

Aspiration Pneumonia—the Big Danger

Every animal's lungs contain thousands of microscopic hollow sacs of cells, the *alveoli*. These sacs are connected by tubes called *bronchi* and *bronchioles* to the animal's *trachea* (windpipe). The sacs become filled with air when the animal inhales and are emptied of air when

the animal exhales. Within the cells of the alveoli, carbon dioxide is exchanged for oxygen in an animal's bloodstream. This exchange of gases is absolutely essential for life.

An animal's trachea and *esophagus* (the tube from the mouth to the stomach) both have entrances into the body inside an animal's mouth. The trachea also has a connected entrance inside the animal's nose. Food gets into the body through the esophagus; air enters the lungs through the trachea.

If a small amount of material other than air enters the trachea by accident, the animal coughs and expels the foreign matter. This is what happens when you swallow food or liquid the wrong way and cough it up. Solid material such as food is usually too large to enter the smaller passages of the lungs that lead to the alveoli. However, liquids can enter these passages and get into even the smallest parts of the lungs.

Liquid-filled alveoli are usually damaged so badly that the cells die. These dead cells in the lungs result in an inflammation of the lung tissue—*pneumonia*.

Air cannot enter alveoli filled with liquids. If enough liquid enters the lungs and causes a large number of alveoli to become nonfunctional, carbon dioxide and oxygen exchange cannot take place. The affected animal dies from lack of oxygen. This is the same as when an animal dies by drowning; fluid fills the lungs.

Every animal, even a newborn, has an automatic reflex that prevents breathing liquids into its lungs when it swallows. However, if liquid is introduced into an animal's mouth too fast or in too large a quantity at one time, the animal cannot swallow it. The liquid will be coughed out, run out of the mouth, or enter the animal's lungs. If a large amount of liquid enters an animal's lungs at once, most of the alveoli become nonfunctional at the same time. The animal drowns just as though it were immersed in water.

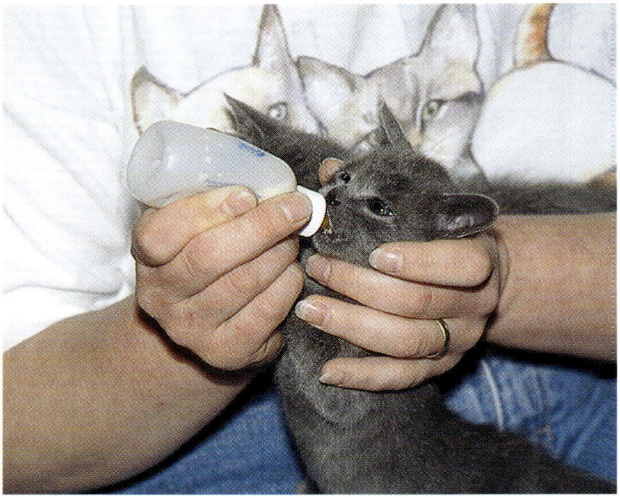

You need to support the kitten's head at first.

If a kitten accidentally gets a little bit of milk into its lungs, it will probably recover. If it gets a considerable amount of milk into its lungs, the kitten will be unable to breathe well. It will become very sick from aspiration pneumonia. If a kitten gets a very large amount of milk into its lungs, as from a stomach tube accidentally placed into the kitten's trachea instead of its esophagus, the kitten will die immediately. It will

actually drown in milk. You must take appropriate precautions to prevent milk formula from entering any of your kittens' lungs.

Using the Pet-Nursing Bottle

When you feed orphaned kittens with a pet-nursing bottle, you must do it properly. The following explains eight factors you must follow to feed the kittens successfully.

Feeding Milk Formula

Fill your bottles with milk formula. Warm the milk by placing the bottles into a cup of hot water for a minute or two. The time-honored method of dropping a little milk onto your wrist will let you feel if the milk is hot enough. The milk should feel very warm; kittens receive warmer milk from their mothers than do human babies. You may need to warm the milk bottle between feeding each kitten. Once your kittens have learned to nurse well from a bottle, the temperature will be of less importance to them. Until they feed well, having the milk at about 102°F (38.9°C) will encourage them to nurse.

The kittens must be in their natural nursing position. When nursing from their mothers, kittens are on their stomachs with their heads extended. They suck on nipples that are horizontal in position. Your kittens will not nurse well if you attempt to hold them on their backs as you would hold a human infant. To make drinking from a bottle as natural as possible for kittens, the kittens should lie on their abdomens on a soft cloth or towel.

Provide warmth to imitate their mother's body heat. Kittens are attracted to their mother's nipples by the odor and warmth of her body. You will not be able to duplicate the mother's odor, but you can supply her warmth. A warm environment will stimulate the kittens to suck. When you feed a kitten, place it onto a heating pad or a warm hot-water bottle that is covered with a towel. The pad or hot-water bottle should be warm to the touch but not hot. The mother cat's body temperature is about 102°F (38.9°C). This is the ideal temperature for your kittens. Place a thermometer onto the towel the first time you feed your kittens. Feel the warmth; you soon will be able to judge by feel if the temperature is acceptable.

Gently introduce the nipple into each kitten's mouth. Before you offer a kitten the bottle, squeeze the plastic nursing bottle just enough so that a drop of milk moistens the nipple. Gently open the kitten's mouth, and stick in the nipple. Stick it all the way in; the presence of the nipple drawn toward the kitten's throat stimulates the sucking reflex. Unlike a mother's nipple attached to flexible skin, the rubber nipple will not extend beyond the plastic rim attaching it to the bottle. This is why you should use as long a nipple as possible and one of appropriate diameter. Move the bottle slightly

back and forth in the kitten's mouth to stimulate it to suck.

Never squeeze the bottle while it is in a kitten's mouth. When you squeeze plastic nursing bottles, milk squirts out. When milk squirts out, a kitten cannot swallow fast enough to prevent milk from accidentally entering its lungs. When milk gets into a kitten's lungs, it may get aspiration pneumonia. If enough milk enters its lungs, it will die. Do not squeeze the bottle while your kittens are nursing.

While they nurse, your kittens may make kneading motions with their front paws. This is the way kittens massage their mother's milk glands to stimulate the release of milk. The motion is entirely normal—even though your kittens are drinking from a bottle, they still have their kneading reflex.

Each kitten should consume its appropriate volume of milk in two or three minutes of sucking. Milk from a bottle comes out much faster than does milk from a mammary gland.

Air must enter the bottle as milk is withdrawn. When a kitten sucks, milk leaves the bottle. This creates a slight vacuum. If this vacuum is not relieved by air entering the bottle, the vacuum soon becomes too strong for the kitten to be able to draw out more milk. Air can enter the bottle in one of two ways:

1. The kitten momentarily loses its sucking action on the nipple, and air enters the bottle around the kitten's tongue, through the hole in the tip of the nipple.

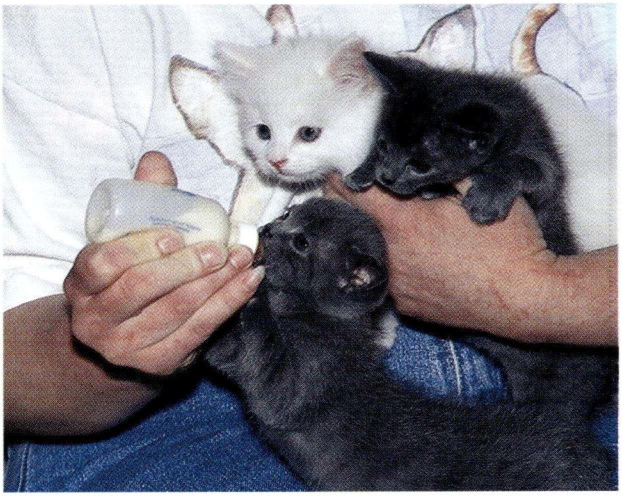

Before long, the kittens will be able to nurse without your support.

2. When the kitten nurses, air is drawn into the bottle around the edge of the cap as the slight vacuum is created.

You should see air bubbles rising in the bottle as milk is withdrawn and air is admitted. If no air bubbles appear, the milk level in the bottle will not go down, and the kitten will not be able to withdraw any milk. If this occurs, check to be sure the hole in the nipple is open and of the correct size. If the nipple appears to be working satisfactorily, turn the plastic collar holding the nipple to the bottle slightly to break the seal and admit a tiny bit of air. If you turn the collar too much, the bottle will leak. If a kitten sucks and sucks and it does not seem to be getting milk, you may have to withdraw the nipple from its mouth, allow air to enter the bottle through the hole in the nipple, then give the nipple back to the kitten.

Milk should not run out of the kitten's mouth. If the kitten drools milk from the corners of its mouth as it nurses, the hole in the nipple is probably too large. The milk is flowing too fast for the kitten to swallow it. Check your equipment, and replace the nipple if necessary.

Be patient—kittens may not learn immediately. A kitten may require a few minutes to learn to suck from a bottle. Move the nipple in and out of the kitten's mouth. This should encourage it to grasp the nipple with its tongue and to suck. If the kitten does not nurse within a few moments, put it back into its bed, feed another kitten, and come back to the first kitten later. Eventually, all reasonably strong kittens will suck on the nipple and consume the milk formula.

Using Stomach Tubes and Syringes

You can feed kittens with a plastic tube passed down their throats and into their stomachs. Doing so takes only seconds to give each kitten its complete meal. Even kittens too weak to nurse from a bottle often can be saved by tube feeding. This technique is not without its drawbacks, however.

- You can accidentally place the feeding tube into a kitten's trachea instead of its esophagus. If you introduce the milk formula into the kitten's lungs instead of its stomach, its lungs will be unable to contain air, and the kitten will surely die.
- The kitten fed with a stomach tube cannot choose the amount of formula it consumes. It receives the volume you introduce into its stomach with the syringe. If you miscalculate or if the kitten's requirements are unusual, you might accidentally underfeed or overfeed it.

Is tube feeding worth the risk? Often, the answer is yes. In the case of very weak kittens, using the feeding tube may be the only way to save them. If you have to hand-feed a large number of kittens, you may not have the time to bottle-feed them all.

If you are careful, you can use the syringe and stomach tube safely.

1. Obtain the correct equipment from your veterinarian.

2. Weigh your kittens, and calculate the amount of formula each needs. The kittens in most litters are almost the same size, so one calculation will be sufficient for all the kittens.

3. Get a veterinarian to demonstrate the procedure. Not all veterinarians have the experience (or the interest) in feeding orphaned kittens by this method. If your veterinarian does not, ask him or her to recommend a colleague who does.

4. Copy the actions of your veterinarian. With the kitten lying in a normal position on its stomach, gently open its mouth with one hand. Insert the tube over the center of its tongue and into its throat. Never

use force; the tube should slide down very easily.

5. Practice passing the stomach tube in the presence of your veterinarian to be sure you are doing it right. You will gain confidence when you see how easy it is.

6. Mark the tube (with an indelible marking pen) at a point just in front of the kitten's nose when the tube is passed down its throat correctly. If the tube will not go down the kitten's throat to the mark, you have not passed it correctly. If this happens, withdraw the tube and pass it again.

7. If the tube will not go down far enough without force, you have probably placed it into the trachea. If you then squirt milk in with the syringe, you will be placing the milk into the kitten's lungs!

The whole procedure sounds frightening. However, after one or two feedings, you will feel like an expert.

- Draw the required amount of milk formula into the syringe.
- Depress the plunger slightly to fill the tube with milk.
- Pass the tube down the kitten's throat.
- Depress the plunger when the tube is in place. Fill the kitten's stomach with the milk formula.
- Be careful not to depress the plunger of the syringe while you are withdrawing it from the kitten's throat. If drops of milk accidentally leak out when the tip of the tube is at the level of the kitten's trachea, the milk may accidentally enter the lungs. If milk remains in the syringe when you withdraw the tube, try to pull the plunger slightly backward to prevent accidental spills.

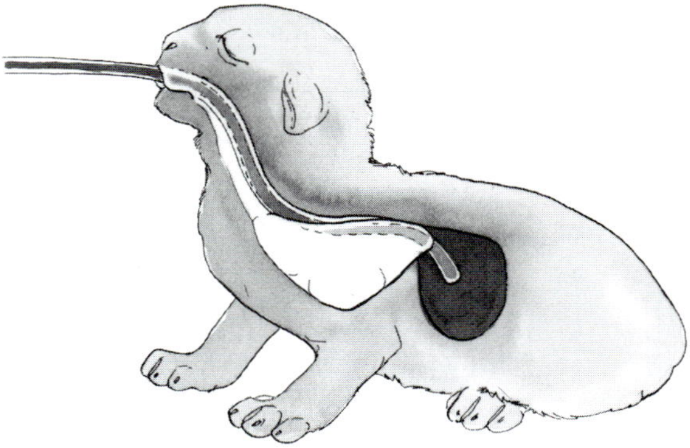

The feeding tube is passed down the throat and into the stomach.

Changing to Bottles

Most people feed orphaned kittens with a bottle if the kittens are normal and strong. If your kittens are weak and you need to use the stomach tube, you can change over to the bottle when the kittens are stronger. Try feeding the kittens with a bottle after a day or two of giving adequate nourishment with a stomach tube. Fill and warm a bottle. Offer it to each kitten. Use the stomach tube for a few more days only for those kittens that are still too weak to suck.

To save time, you can continue feeding your kittens with the tube until they have opened their eyes. When their eyes are open, kittens will become too active to pass the tube easily unless you have had a lot of practice.

Chapter Seven
Weaning the Kittens

If a mother cat continues to produce milk, her kittens will continue to nurse until they are at least 12 weeks of age. Kittens raised by their mothers will start to show interest in her food when they are about five weeks old. By three months, kittens that are still with the queen may nurse occasionally but will obtain most of their nutrient requirements from solid food. By four months, most kittens have lost their sucking reflex, and most queens have stopped lactating (producing milk). A few kittens and cats continue to nurse into adulthood—some cats nurse on inanimate objects (wool sucking, for example) throughout their lives. Research has not proven that early weaning has an influence on the continuation of the sucking behavior past nursing age.

How to Wean Your Kittens

You should not plan to bottle-feed your kittens for as long a time as a mother cat would nurse her litter. No matter how good the formula you use, you cannot provide milk that is as nutritious as their mother's milk. In addition, you cannot feed your kittens as often (every hour or two) as does a mother cat. Your kittens should obtain at least part of their nutrition from solid food as soon as possible.

Kittens, puppies, and human babies are able to swallow food before they are physically able to eat by themselves. Human children are started on spoon-fed cereal and other foods before they can physically convey the food to their mouths. Your kittens will be able to swallow solid food before they can take it from a dish.

Your kittens should be weaned gradually. If your kittens were with their mother, they would experiment with eating her food around the age of five weeks. At this age, they would still be receiving the majority of their nutrients from their mother's milk. By the time they were eight or ten weeks old, they would be eating a significant amount of solid food and receiving only a small percentage of their nutrition from nursing.

Do not stop bottle-feeding your orphans when you start giving them a diet containing solid foods. At

each feeding, first offer the solid food, then the bottle. If the kittens' stomachs are filled with solids, they will drink relatively little milk formula. Their nutritional level will be raised by eating the solid food—queens' milk is about 75 percent water.

Start feeding solid food when your kittens are four weeks of age. Hold a tiny piece of food to a kitten's lips. Allow it to smell the food, then gently place the morsel into the kitten's mouth. Wait a moment for it to swallow, then offer another bite. Once it has learned to expect a bit of food, the kitten will readily take it from your fingers.

At four weeks, your kittens should accept about one-half to one teaspoonful of food before you offer it the bottle that contains its usual formula. Check to be sure the kitten has swallowed each bit of food before you offer another. Never cram a kitten's mouth full of unswallowed food.

When your kittens are five weeks old, they will be physically able to eat bits of food from a plate. Offer the food on a plate, not in a bowl. Each kitten can then pick up pieces of the food without the necessity of reaching over the rim of a bowl. You can use a paper plate or a piece of newspaper on which to feed your kittens, then discard the leftovers with the plate. If you are feeding more than five kittens, you may need to offer the litter two plates of food to be sure each kitten can get its share. Expect the kittens to walk all over the food at first. You might have to wipe food off their paws after they have eaten.

House Your Kittens Together

When your kittens are able to take food from a plate, you can leave food in their enclosures so that they can eat whenever they are hungry. At this time you can house the littermates as a group instead of each in its own box.

For this, you need a cage or some sort of escape-proof enclosure. When your kittens are a little older, you can keep them together in a small room such as a bathroom, with the toilet lid down. At first, you can keep them in a huge cardboard box. Remember, kittens are good at jumping up and catching the top of a box with their paws. If they can get to the top, they can get out of the box.

Take the dividers out of one of your kitten boxes to make a bed big enough for all the kittens at once. Cut the side off the box to enable the kittens to go in and out with ease. Line the bed with some of the old bedding from two or more of the kittens; they will recognize their own smells. Place this bed inside your cage; add the kittens at mealtime.

Give them a plate of food to keep them busy. Feed the kittens often, a small amount at one time. Soon they will forget about sucking and look forward to their meals on a plate.

If your kittens persist in sucking on each other, you have put them

together too soon. This will not likely happen once they can eat from a plate. However, if it does, feed them more often, and offer some food that they really love.

What to Feed Your Kittens

Encourage your kittens to eat by feeding what they crave. Forget feeding cereal and milk or even cat food mixtures. Kittens are able to pick up and eat pieces of solid food before they can learn to lap gruel. Even though kittens may walk on their solid food at first, they stay much cleaner than they will in the future when they wade through puddles of semiliquid preparations.

If the odor of the food is really enticing, even very young kittens will make the effort to eat it. What is a wild cat's normal prey? What does a wild feline catch to feed her young? Certainly not a mushy cereal-and-milk mixture; she feeds her kittens meat!

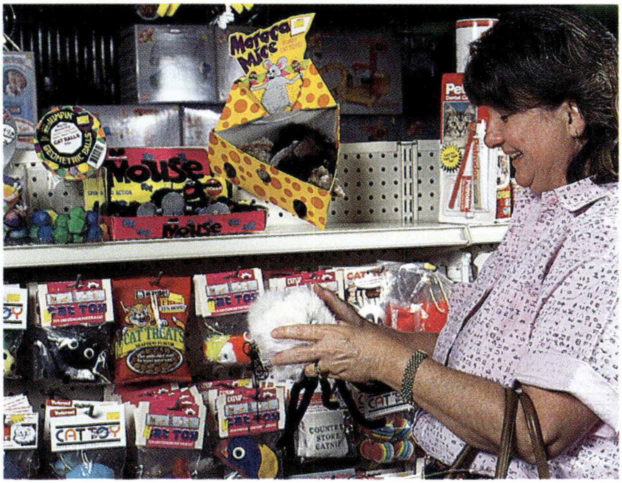

You can choose from many kinds of commercial foods.

No, do not catch and feed your kittens mice to wean them. Just go to the grocery store and buy some nice, freshly ground beef. Cook the meat thoroughly, allow it to cool, and crumble it into small pieces. Offer a tiny pinch of the well-cooked ground meat to a kitten and see what happens. Often, the kitten will bite your finger in its eagerness to eat. When it can walk and run well (at about five weeks old), it will be happy to feed itself.

Provide a Complete Diet

Meat alone is not an adequate diet for kittens. After no more than two days of feeding meat, start mixing some high-quality kitten food with it. Within three or four meals, eliminate the meat altogether, and feed only regular kitten growth diet. The kittens will have learned to anticipate a delicious meal and will eat even though you are not feeding them meat.

Feed canned kitten food or dry kitten food that you have soaked until it is soft. Soak the dry food in water, not milk or formula. Always refrigerate uneaten portions until the next feeding.

Commercial premium brands of dry food intended for kittens contain about 35 percent protein, 20 percent fat, and no more than 10 percent moisture. Canned food contains about 10 percent protein, 2.5 percent fat, and about 80 percent moisture. When you buy canned food,

you are paying more for water and processing than you are when you buy dry kitten food.

A convenient method of feeding is to use soaked dry kitten food to which you have added about 25 percent canned meat-type cat food. This addition will only slightly increase the protein content of the diet but will greatly increase the diet's palatability.

Feed Several Meals a Day

Offer food to your kittens every six or eight hours. Allow them to eat their fill. After 30 minutes, remove and discard or refrigerate the left-overs. Do not leave moist food in the kittens' pen; it will spoil rapidly. You will soon learn just how much your kittens will eat. Remember, though, they are growing rapidly, and their requirements are also growing.

Food right out of the refrigerator will not harm your orphans. However, they might prefer it warmed, especially when they are just starting to eat solids.

At age six to eight weeks, kittens will be able to chew up pieces of dry food. You can keep a small bowl of dry meal in their pen for snacks. Select a kitten food that comes in small, easy-to-chew pieces.

Provide Fresh Water

Once you have eliminated bottle-feeding, you need to provide your kittens with a pan of fresh water. If their bodies require it, their instinct will show them how to drink it. Use a shallow pan that is hard to tip.

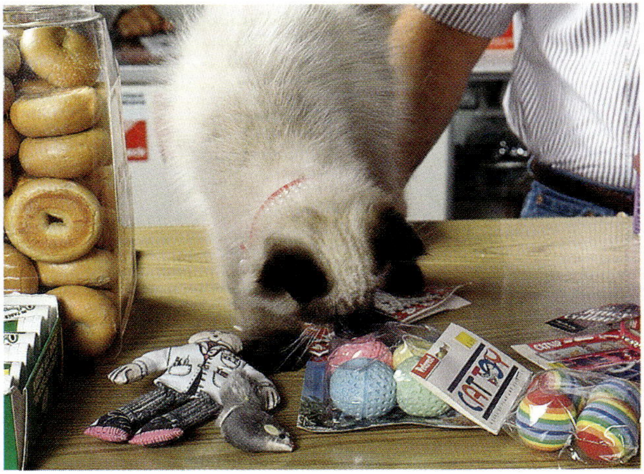

Read the labels and select the best food for your kittens.

Do not worry if your kittens seem to consume very little water. Their diet, even if it consists largely of soaked kitten meal, contains about 70 percent moisture. If they need water, they will drink it.

Do Not Overfeed

Kittens gain approximately a pound a month from birth to five or six months of age. Your orphaned kittens will undoubtedly be smaller

Eliminating the Bottles
By the time a normal kitten is six weeks old, you do not need to feed it with a bottle. Almost all six-week-old kittens will have been weaned for ten days or more. If your kittens do not eat well, go back to the plain ground meat for a day or two. Put your bottles away for the next litter of orphaned kittens.

A six-week-old kitten can eat commercial food.

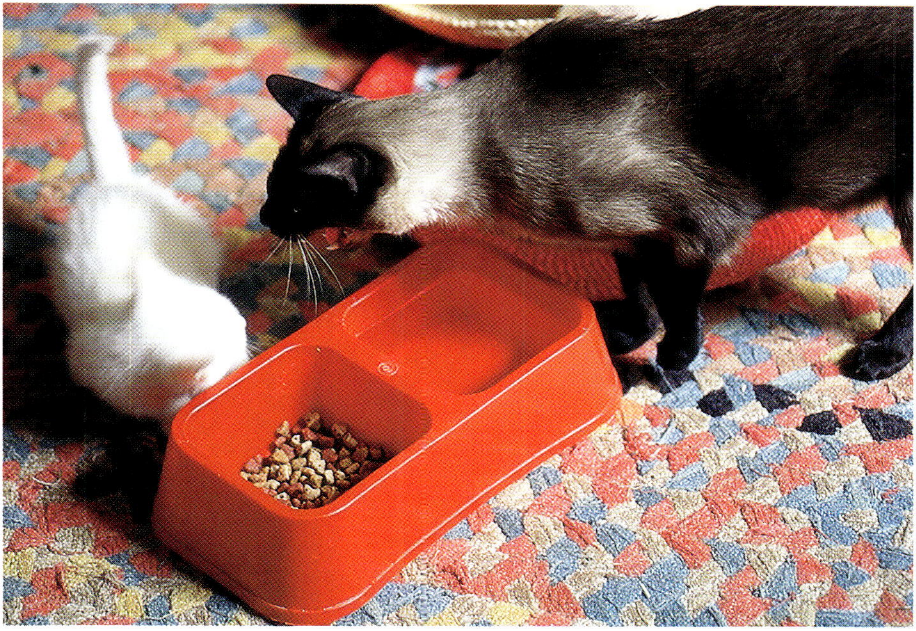

at four weeks than they would if a healthy queen raised them. No matter how hard you try, you cannot supply the nutrients to orphans that nature supplies through their natural mothers. At eight weeks, your orphans should have caught up in weight to all but the largest queen-raised kittens because you can supply them with a diet that provides adequate nutrition for growth. Excellent commercial cat and kitten foods are available in every grocery store. Selecting those feeds that have undergone the feeding trials of the Association of American Feed Control Officials (AAFCO) is important. Select only feeds that have been found to provide "complete and balanced nutrition for all stages of life." If the feed is so tested and certified, this statement will appear on the bag or can.

How do you know if you are feeding the correct amount?

1. Your kittens should clean up nearly all the food offered within 30 minutes. If they leave much food on their plate, offer less at the next feeding.

2. The kittens should be eager for their next meal. Overfed kittens tend to ignore their food. If your kittens are not ready and waiting for you to bring their food, try feeding less or feeding less often. Maybe your kittens need only three meals a day, not four.

3. The kittens should appear plump and active. They should grow constantly but not at a constant rate. Kittens, like other babies, have

growth spurts and periods of little gain. Weigh your kittens weekly. If any of them fail to gain at least a couple of ounces in a week, try to determine the reason. A common reason for failure to gain is failure to compete with littermates—the largest kittens may push the smallest ones away from the plate. Separate your kittens, or feed from two or more plates.

4. Your kittens should have formed stools. Loose, watery stools indicate that something has gone wrong.

Diarrhea in Kittens

The color of kittens' stools is not very important, but the form of the stools is important. Almost all commercial feeds contain dyes that produce a uniform color throughout the product. These dyes will affect the color of your kittens' stools but not the form.

Unformed stools can range in consistency from merely soft to completely liquid. In cases of severe or prolonged diarrhea, liquid stools might contain blood. Consider any stool that does not keep its shape to be diarrhea.

Diarrhea in otherwise healthy kittens usually has one of two causes: overfeeding or internal parasites. If your kittens have unformed stools but are playful and eager to eat, try these remedies. Try all three remedies at the same time.

Feed less for a few meals. Give only two-thirds the usual amount of food to your kittens. If their stools have not formed within 24 hours, overfeeding is not the cause. If the stools become formed, increase the kittens' feed very gradually.

Feed low-bulk, easily digested food for 24 hours. Give your kittens a mixture of one-half ground beef and one-half boiled rice. Mix these together very well so that the kittens cannot pick out the meat and leave the rice. You need not change to this mixture gradually. If your kittens have runny stools, remove their regular food, and give them beef and rice.

Have stool samples examined. Take a sample of several of the kittens' stools to your veterinarian to be examined under the microscope for evidence of internal parasites. When you collect the sample to take to the veterinarian, use a tongue depressor or a disposable plastic spoon to gather a small amount of several stools. Select portions of stools from more than one kitten.

Weigh your kittens to enable your veterinarian to dispense medication in an appropriate dose if he or she finds parasite eggs in the stools. If the stools are negative for parasites, wait two weeks and have another composite stool sample of the litter examined. If the kittens' stools remain loose and you have tried all the remedies, make an appointment to take the entire litter to your veterinarian for a checkup.

Chapter Eight

Socializing Orphaned Kittens

A cat's mental health is as important as its physical health. The aim is to ensure that hand-raised kittens grow up to be comfortable and secure in a society of humans and other animals.

The kitten raised by humans has an entirely different start in life than one raised by a mother cat. The hand-raised kitten is kept in isolation from its littermates for the first three weeks of its life. Its human caretaker provides food only at intervals. The caretaker, not the queen, also provides warmth and sanitation. No wonder hand-raised kittens may be different mentally as well as physically than kittens raised by their mothers.

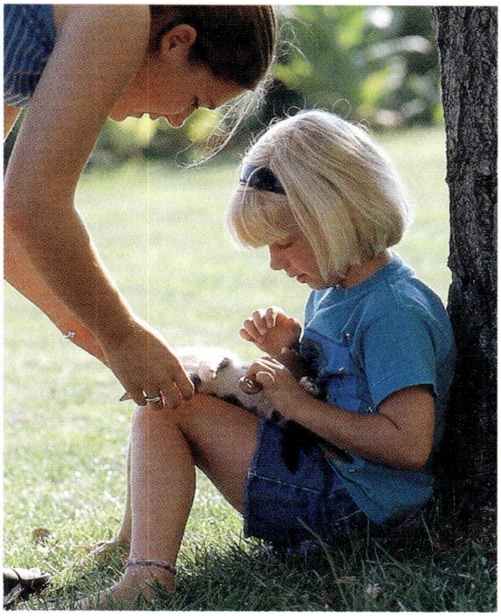

Your kittens should meet many people.

When you raise a newborn kitten, you have the opportunity and the responsibility to help it develop behaviors that will make it a friendly, cooperative pet. The kitten's entire life is literally in your hands.

Handling Your Kittens

Some have suggested that kittens raised in isolation from other kittens may become cats that are more frightened by strange people, strange animals, and new places than are kittens raised with their siblings. Since hand-raised kittens are housed with their littermates after they are weaned, this is not an important consideration. From the

age of three or four weeks, hand-raised kittens interact with each other to the same degree as kittens raised by a queen.

Hand-raised kittens may have a greater potential to become affectionate, cooperative pets than kittens that have little human contact until they are weaned. How do you want your pet cat to act?

- Your pet cat should show affection toward you and members of your family.
- Your cat should use its litter box dependably and never urinate or defecate in other places in your house.
- Your cat should never bite or scratch any person or other animal without extreme provocation.
- Your cat should accept visitors in your home without hissing or hiding.
- Your cat should allow you to cut its nails, comb it, brush it, and give it oral medication without any sign of resistance.
- Your veterinarian should be able to examine your cat, look into its mouth, clean its ears, and even give it injections without a struggle.
- Traveling in a carrier should not be stressful or terrifying to your cat.
- Your cat should respect your authority and stay off forbidden places such as kitchen counters.

Sounds too good to be true? When you raise a kitten by hand, you have the opportunity to create a perfect pet. The kittens that you keep will be delightful companions. The kittens that you place into other homes will be valued by their owners.

Housing Weaned Kittens

When they are able to eat by themselves, at 21 to 28 days of age, you should house your litter of kittens together. They need a large cage or enclosure from which they cannot escape and then wander into danger or away from their source of food. An enclosure of about 2-by-3 feet (0.6-by-1 m) in size is adequate until the kittens are eight or nine weeks of age and ready to go to their permanent homes.

The most convenient type of enclosure for a litter of kittens is a wire cage with a top and a secure door. A large wire dog cage is ideal if the spacing between the wires is too small to allow the kittens to escape. If you do not have a cage, you can use a large cardboard carton temporarily. However, you will need to replace the carton when it becomes wet and dirty. If you use a solid-sided box, place it under a window where the kittens can get plenty of light.

Kittens are very active jumpers and climbers. Unless your box is very deep, the kittens will learn to climb out. If your box is deep enough to contain the kittens, it will be inconvenient for you to reach the bottom to handle the kittens and clean the litter box. If you improvise a lid for a box with a couple of window screens or some similar material, fasten the lid to the box so a climbing kitten cannot dislodge it.

As they grow, the kittens will interact with each other, begin to initiate play behavior, and compete for food.

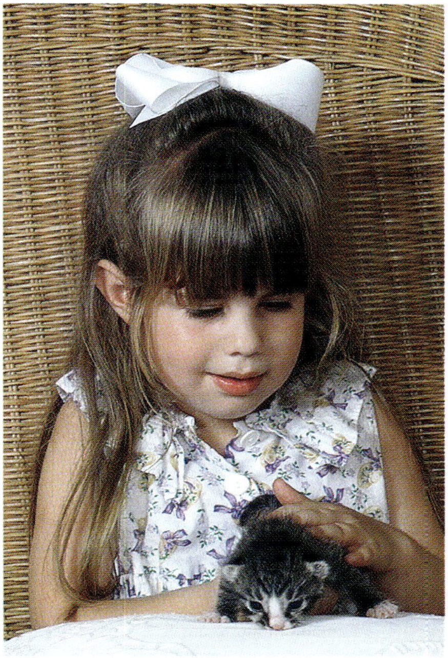

The little girl is holding the kitten on a pillow for its safety.

It is important that you provide enough space at the food plates so that none of the kittens will be crowded out by the others. Use several food plates for large litters.

Alternate Feeding Locations

Kittens need human socialization as well as littermate socialization if they are to develop into trusting pets. The time to socialize hand-raised kittens is when they are fed.

During the first few days that kittens are housed together and are eating by themselves, place the food plates inside their cage, allow them to eat all they will, then remove the leftovers. When the kittens eagerly rush to the plates, select one mealtime when you have the leisure to take the kittens out of their cage and feed them in a different location. Carry the kittens to another room in the house, and offer the food when they are hungry. If they are more interested in exploring the new area, allow them to look around until the smell of their dinner entices them. Return them to the cage after they have eaten. If the kittens do not eat as much in a new location as they did in their cage, place the plates into the cage, and let them finish their meal.

If you have a litter of six or more kittens, divide the litter, and feed half the kittens in the cage and half in another room. Alternate the feeding locations for each kitten every day. When the kittens are comfortable enough in every location to eat hungrily when food is provided, you need not continue to feed them in different places.

Alternate Handlers

Do not be your kittens' only handler. Allow them to become acquainted with as many people and places as possible. Be sure that each experience is pleasant for the kittens. Carry them gently, place them down onto the floor carefully, and speak to them before you pick them up to avoid startling them.

Do not try to carry more than one kitten in each hand, or you may have to squeeze them to keep from dropping one. If a child carries a kitten, wrap the kitten in a folded towel in the child's hands. The kitten will cling with its claws to the towel and not accidentally scratch the child in

an attempt to secure a grasp. When children are scratched, they tend to drop and frighten or injure kittens.

Visiting Friends

Nothing is wrong with taking your kittens to a friend's house for a short visit, to your child's classroom for show-and-tell, or to the backyard for a play session. Protect your kittens from exposure to diseases and parasites by taking them only to locations without other cats.

Take the kittens in a carrier lined with a towel or newspapers. Take some of their food along to feed them in a new location.

If you have a large litter, take only two or three kittens at a time, and alternate the ones that get to go. Start taking the kittens on little visits when they are six weeks of age—they will be old enough to benefit from the experience. While you are teaching your kittens to be at home in new places, you will also be teaching them to ride in a carrier without fear or resentment.

Small kittens tire very easily. After the kittens have played, explored, and eaten in the new place, put them back into the carrier for a rest. Taking kittens home to their own cages (and litter boxes) soon after they are fed is best. Take clean newspapers along, just in case you do not get them home in time.

Of course, watch to be sure that everyone handles your kittens gently. Have small children sit on the floor and hold the kittens in their laps. That way, the kittens cannot accidentally be dropped or jump out of the children's hands.

Take your kittens to visit children only after the kittens have received sufficient and appropriate veterinary care. You must be positive that the kittens have no parasites transmissible to humans. Supervise the children washing their hands after they have handled the kittens. Chapter 11 details the health problems that may exist between kittens and humans.

Raising a Single Kitten

A single hand-raised kitten has no littermates; you will have to provide all of its social contacts yourself. Feeding a single kitten in several places, having numerous people handle the kitten, and allowing it to explore locations other than its box or cage are particularly important. If you have other cats or dogs that will not harm a kitten, you should introduce your kitten to them when it is three to six weeks of age. Be sure that the kitten has no parasites before you allow another animal to lick it.

Grooming Your Kittens

Both queen-raised and human-raised kittens have been stimulated to urinate and defecate before they were able to carry out these reflex actions by themselves. Kittens raised by their mothers have been licked all over. However, hand-raised kittens often get no other

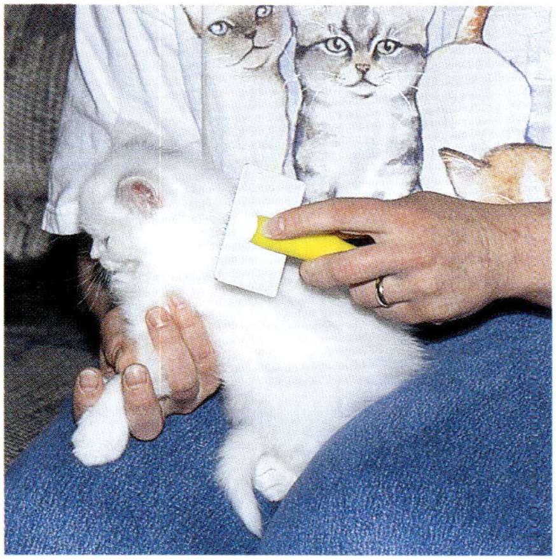

Teach your kittens to be groomed with a slicker brush.

grooming from their handlers unless they get filthy and need a bath.

The time to teach kittens to tolerate grooming is when they are tiny. If properly trained, your kittens will submit to combing, brushing, and nail trimming for their entire lives. If a kitten is properly trained to tolerate grooming when it is small, brushing out its dead hair, clipping off its mats, and cutting its nails will be easy. Its owner's house will not be full of cat hair and clawed furniture. Its veterinarian will love your trained kitten when it offers no resistance to examination or injections.

Start grooming your kittens when their eyes are open. Since even Persian kittens have short coats at birth, you will have to do little actual grooming. You are merely teaching your kittens to offer no resistance to the process of grooming as well as to any other kind of nonpainful handling.

You will need a metal comb with about 12 teeth to the inch for shorthaired kittens. If your kittens will be longhaired, get the kind of comb that has a coarse end with 6 teeth to the inch and a fine end with 12. Buy a metal comb. Human hard-rubber combs generate too much static electricity and may be uncomfortable for your kittens.

The actual grooming of a small kitten is simple. Place the kitten onto a folded towel to make it feel secure. Gently comb through the hair on its back, neck, and hind legs with the fine end of your comb. Then turn it over, and gently comb its belly and throat. You will remove little if any loose hair; your aim is to train the kitten to tolerate the handling. Groom each kitten for about a minute, two or three times a week, from the time its eyes open. The kitten is most likely to struggle when you turn it onto its back. Ignore it. Do not punish it, shake it, or yell at it. Hold the kitten down, and continue grooming. That is what its mother would do.

Trimming Nails

Trim your kittens' nails at each grooming session. Very young kittens' nails do not yet retract. For older kittens, gently press each tiny paw until the nails are exposed. Snip only the very tips of each nail with a human nail trimmer held at right angles to the kitten's toe. Actually snip each nail only once every week or two; kittens' nails do not grow very fast. During the other grooming sessions, go through the motions, but do not cut anything off the nails. Allow the kitten to become accustomed to the procedure.

Use a sharp human fingernail trimmer, not a dog or cat nail cutter, because snipping off only the tiny tip of the nail is easy with a human trimmer. A human fingernail trimmer will work well on all but the largest adult cat nails. A human toenail trimmer will cut even those more safely, quickly, and inexpensively than will a trimmer made for cats. When the human trimmers get dull, they are cheap enough to discard and buy a new sharp one.

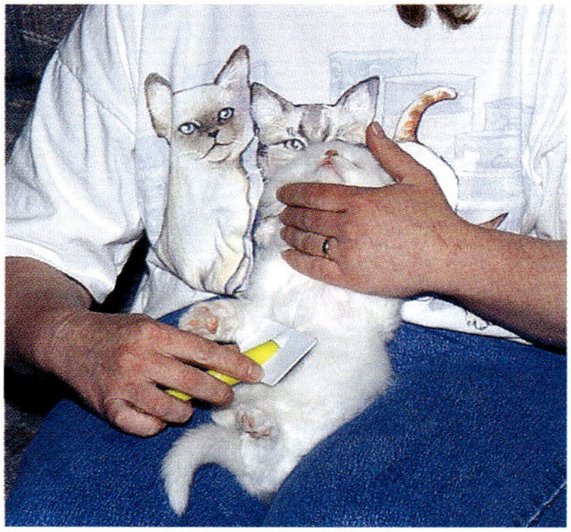

Be sure to brush the tummy as well as the back.

Bathing

Your kittens will rarely need a bath. Only if they become filthy will you wash an entire kitten. You can easily clean most messes off kittens with a piece of damp cotton or a moistened cloth. Be sure to use warm water and to keep wet kittens in a warm place until they are dry.

If you must bathe the kittens, wash one at a time. Swish it around in a small basin of tepid water. Keep its head above water at all times. Rub the soiled areas with a piece of cotton. Change the water when it becomes dirty. If you cannot remove all the dirt with cotton, comb through the kitten's hair with the fine end of your metal comb. Wipe the kitten with clean towels, and keep it warm until it has completely dried. If you must use soap, use only the mildest baby shampoo you can find.

You may have to bathe kittens if they have fleas. Do not use flea shampoo; it is too toxic to use on kittens less than a month old. Dampen each kitten with warm water, and comb the fleas out of the coat with a fine-tooth comb. Fleas will escape the wider teeth of a regular metal cat comb. Fine-tooth combs are available at drugstores or at pet stores, where they are sold as *flea combs*. As you remove fleas from a kitten, rinse the comb in a bowl of soapy water to drown the fleas caught in the teeth.

Litter Box Training

Cats instinctively bury their eliminations. Outdoor cats scratch a shallow depression in the ground, eliminate in the depression, then paw the loose soil over their urine and feces. Unless they are scent-marking, outdoor cats seldom use the same spot twice. Cats prefer to eliminate in clean places.

Indoor cats are supposed to do the same thing in their litter boxes: scrape away some litter, eliminate, then scratch litter over their excrement. Most indoor cats comply with this arrangement, but cats are fussy.

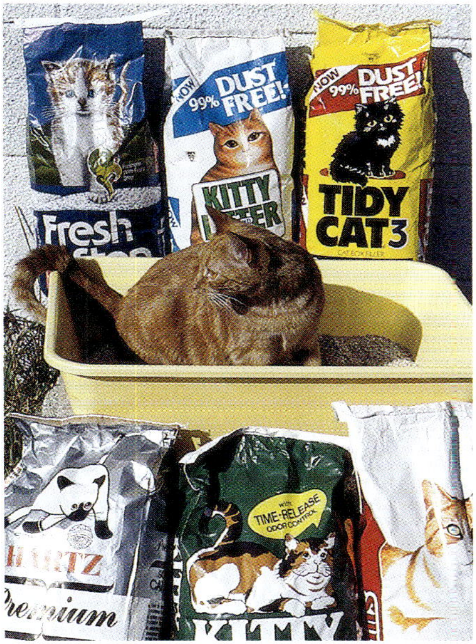

Start with plain clay litter and switch to other types only when your kitten has learned to use its box.

They dislike using a dirty litter box, and will often choose another place to eliminate if their boxes are not kept clean. Indoor cats can develop a preference for certain litter box fillers—plain clay litter, torn newspapers, clumping litter—and refuse to use a box filled with other substances. Unfortunately, indoor cats can develop a preference for eliminating on unacceptable surfaces, such as carpeting. Prevent bad habits before they start. Train your hand-raised kittens to have acceptable elimination behavior.

No, kittens do not learn to use a litter box by watching their mothers. They instinctively use their mother's litter box because that is where they smell their mother's excrement. Use this instinct to train your motherless kittens to use their own box.

When you first house your kittens together, they will eliminate almost anywhere in the enclosure. You will need to change the newspapers and bedding several times a day to keep the area clean. Within a day or two, you will notice that the kittens have selected one place for most of their excrement. At first, the kittens may not always eliminate only in this place, and the place may change from day to day.

By the time the kittens are five weeks old, they will be more consistent in eliminating in one area. This is the time to introduce the litter box. Get a box with sides no more than 2 inches (5 cm) high. Plastic cat litter boxes are often too deep for small kittens to learn to use. A cardboard box cut to the correct height is satisfactory, even though you will need to replace it frequently. Line the litter box with newspapers, and place it over the spot the kittens have selected as their bathroom. Take some of the papers on which the kittens have already eliminated, and put the dirty papers into the box to establish the *right* smell. You need not put commercial cat litter into the box at this time. Your kittens will have learned to eliminate on the newspapers in their cage. At four to five weeks of age, they will have no idea about the purpose of litter.

Kittens often select new areas in which they choose to eliminate. You may need to move the litter box location or use more than one litter box within the kittens' enclosure until they establish habits. If the kit-

tens tend to displace the litter box as they play in the enclosure, fasten the box to the sides of the enclosure with a couple of clothespins.

Change the papers in the litter box frequently to prevent the kittens from seeking a cleaner spot in which to eliminate. The size of the litter will determine how often the box should be changed. A single kitten will need its box cleaned daily; a litter of four will need its box changed at least twice a day.

To clean the litter box, dump the dirty papers into the trash, then reline the box with fresh newspapers. During the first few days, do not clean the box completely. Leave a piece of dirty paper to encourage the kittens to return to the box to eliminate.

Kittens do not develop the dig-and-bury elimination behavior until they are six to eight weeks old. Until that age, they use their litter box merely because they are habituated to the location and the smell. The mere presence of litter will not encourage them to use a litter box. At about six weeks of age, you will see your kittens start to scratch the papers in the litter box before they eliminate and then scratch again after they have finished. If you wish to train them to use litter, start with plain clay litter, and place only a small amount on top of the newspapers. Gradually add more litter each day until you have filled the box to a depth of 1 inch (2 cm).

Commercial Litter

With proper conditioning, cats can be habituated to eliminate on whatever surface their owners choose, not just in a substance in which they can dig. Decide if you want to train your kittens to use litter or just newspapers in their litter box. Litter must be specially purchased; litter can be tracked all over the house; used litter may be more difficult to dispose of. Newspapers are inexpensive; newspapers cannot be tracked through the house; newspapers are easily discarded in the trash. However, some cat litters are scented to control odors, and buried feces are less unattractive than feces on newspaper. Cat litter requires less-frequent cleaning than newspapers. You can scoop solid waste out of cat litter, while you must completely replace newspapers. If you do not use litter in your cat boxes, your cats will still go through the dig-and-bury procedure without actually digging or burying their eliminations. If you would rather your cats buried their feces, you can place shredded newspaper on top of the folded paper in the boxes.

When your kittens go to their permanent homes, give each new owner a plastic freezer bag containing some of the slightly dirty contents of the litter box the kittens had been using. Instruct each owner to pour the contents of the plastic bag on top of the kittens' new litter and to keep the kittens confined so that they can find their new box easily. The kittens will establish correct elimination behavior within a few days in their new homes.

Chapter Nine

Your Kittens' Perinatal Health

Peri means *around;* natal means *birth.* Perinatal health includes all the medical considerations of kittens from late gestation through the first months of their lives.

Orphaned kittens are at a very significant disadvantage for three reasons:

1. Many orphaned kittens have not received colostrum, the first milk produced by the queen. Colostrum contains many substances that contribute to kittens' immunity to disease for the first two or three months of their lives. Kittens that have nursed from their birth mothers for the first two days of their lives have a greater chance to resist certain bacterial and viral conditions. Kittens that have never nursed from their birth mothers may succumb to infections that would not affect queen-raised kittens.

2. Abandoned orphaned kittens may have suffered starvation and chilling before they were rescued. They may have damage to their intestinal and respiratory systems that is difficult to overcome.

3. Even the best care provided by a human cannot equal the care provided by the kittens' own mother. Hand-raised kittens will be smaller at weaning than their queen-raised counterparts. If you can keep your kittens growing and developing until they are able to eat solid food, they will catch up to kittens that enjoyed the ideal diet and the constant attention of their birth mothers.

You must keep orphaned kittens warm, clean, and fed if they are to have any chance of survival. When you adopt orphaned kittens, your first responsibility is to provide the necessities to keep them alive. After you have fed and housed your kittens adequately, determine what other steps are necessary to keep them thriving.

Examining for Birth Defects

Few kittens are born with *congenital* (present at birth) defects. Some birth defects are obvious, such as a

missing limb. Some are hidden, such as a defective heart. Other defects can be found only if you inspect your kittens with great care.

Some birth defects are life threatening, some are relatively minor. If you are unlucky enough to adopt newborn kittens with birth defects, you must make this decision: should these kittens be euthanized immediately? Your veterinarian can help you decide.

Inherited defects result from the action of genes from one or both parents. An animal may be a carrier of a defect but appear to be normal. If that animal mates with an animal with the same genetic defect, their offspring may inherit defective genes from both their mother and their father. Such animals will probably have the genetic defect.

Some defects are present at birth but do not result from defective genes. These defects are caused by an accident during fetal development or the exposure of a pregnant queen to a *teratogen,* a substance that can cause birth defects.

Kittens with birth defects are often absorbed during fetal development, miscarried, or born dead. Others die soon after birth.

Congenital Defects

No congenital defects commonly occur in the cat. Some conditions occur occasionally.

Cleft Palate. A cleft palate is a longitudinal slitlike opening in the roof of the mouth. This opening communicates with the nasal cavity. When an animal with a cleft palate nurses, the milk may come out of its nose instead of being swallowed down its throat. Milk in the animal's nasal cavity may enter its lungs, resulting in aspiration pneumonia. Depending on the size of the cleft, the affected animal may be hardly affected or unable to nurse at all.

Gently open your kittens' mouths and examine the roof. They should not have any slitlike opening. If the kittens have a large cleft, it will be obvious to you. Occasionally a cleft lip accompanies a cleft palate. A cleft lip is also known as a harelip and should be easy to see. If you have doubts, ask your veterinarian to examine the kittens.

Kittens with cleft palates can be raised by feeding them with a tube. The milk is placed directly into their

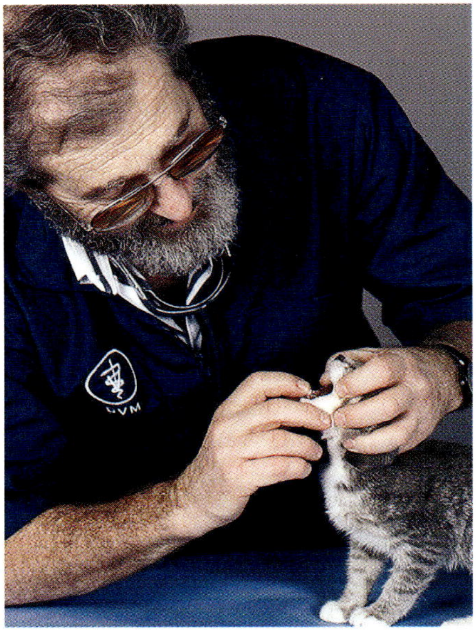

Your kitten needs regular veterinary checkups.

stomachs and bypasses the cleft entirely. Give careful thought to raising these kittens, however. When they are weaned, they may be unable to eat and drink normally. Surgery to correct cleft palate in kittens is difficult and expensive.

Improperly Formed Intestinal Tract. The most common defect of the intestinal tract is a missing portion. Affected kittens may appear normal at birth but soon are sick. Many of these kittens have an undeveloped anus and do not defecate. Some of these kittens die without any apparent cause. Only an autopsy will show what went wrong. Defects of a kitten's intestinal tract are even less common than cleft palates.

Hydrocephalus. This means *water on the brain,* the same condition that occasionally affects human and other infant animals. Hydrocephalus results from a failure of normal fluid drainage to the brain. It is treated surgically only in human infants. Severely affected kittens will die.

Heart Defects. Kittens with severely defective hearts will not live. Kittens with minor defects may appear normal until they are weaned. After weaning, they may be stunted, weak, and listless. Your veterinarian may be able to detect significant heart defects by listening to a kitten's chest with a stethoscope.

Polydactyly (Many Toes). Many kittens are born with two or more extra toes on each front foot or one or more extra toes on each back foot. Cat fanciers call these *mitten paws*. Polydactyly is entirely harmless to affected kittens and even desirable to some owners. Kittens with mitten paws may be more desired when you try to find new homes for them.

Tailless. Manx cats are born with kinked tails, stubbed tails, or no tails. This is an inherited trait in the breed and a common genetic trait in mixed-breed cats. Like mitten paws, many owners favor taillessness. Some kittens that inherit a tailless gene from each parent will not live. However, most are unaffected by the condition.

Teratogens That Can Cause Birth Defects

Griseofulvin is a drug often used to treat ringworm in cats. Griseofulvin may cause severe birth defects if pregnant queens receive it. The defects are usually very obvious, and the affected kittens do not live.

Griseofulvin is often administered to purebred cats in catteries where ringworm is common. It is not likely that you will unknowingly adopt a kitten with defects induced by this drug.

Viral Disease. The exposure of a pregnant queen to feline viral disease may result in her kittens being born with *cerebellar hypoplasia*. This is a condition in which a portion of the brain (the *cerebellum*) is underdeveloped (*hypoplasia*).

In certain respects, cerebellar hypoplasia in kittens resembles cerebral palsy in humans, although the diseases do not affect the same part of the brain. Kittens with cerebellar hypoplasia appear normal until weaning. When affected kittens are old

enough to walk, those with cerebellar hypoplasia will be very shaky and clumsy. Some of them will appear to be unable to eat and drink unaided.

Not every kitten in a litter of an exposed queen will be affected. Both normal kittens and *ataxic* (uncoordinated) kittens may be in the same litter. Not every kitten with the condition will be affected to the same degree. Some will be very shaky; some will hardly be affected at all.

Kittens that are not severely affected with cerebellar hypoplasia can be taught to eat by offering them something that they really want and that they can grasp easily: small pieces of meat! Once they are eating, these kittens can be gradually changed over to cat food. They will learn to lap water and will even learn to eat dry food.

Cats with cerebellar hypoplasia have entirely normal intelligence. Only their motor skills are affected. Cerebellar hypoplastic cats can make great pets: they cannot jump onto kitchen counters. They are usually not able to scratch furniture and never need to be declawed. Give affected cats shallow litter boxes so they can get into them without difficulty. These ataxic cats must never be allowed outdoors, as they cannot climb trees or run away from danger.

Diseases Occurring After Birth

If kittens have had any contact with their mother immediately after birth, they might have caught some diseases. This is true even if the contact the kittens had with their birth mother was less than a few hours in length.

Ascarids. Kittens that have nursed from their mother have a huge advantage: they received colostrum, their mother's first milk. This milk contains essential antibodies that kittens can absorb for only their first few hours and that help protect the kittens from disease.

Kittens that have nursed from their mother also have a disadvantage. They may have ingested the eggs of the cat roundworm. These eggs will develop in the kittens' intestines and make it necessary that the kittens be treated for roundworms around the time they are weaned. Whether or not your kittens have nursed, you should have them checked for roundworms and treated if necessary.

Ringworm. If the queen was affected with ringworm, even if she had no lesions (sores), the kittens are likely to develop ringworm when they are two or three months of age. This is true even if the kittens had only a very limited contact with the queen after they were born.

When you adopt newborn kittens, you seldom know if the queen was carrying the ringworm organism or if your kittens will develop the condition later. The possibility of ringworm is not a reason to avoid hand-raising orphaned kittens, but it is reason to take special precautions.

If you notice any suspicious hairless patches on your kittens, ask your veterinarian to conduct the

Chapter 11 explains the dangers of some diseases shared by humans and cats.

appropriate tests to determine if the condition is caused by ringworm.

Rabies. Veterinarians do not know for certain if a mother cat that has been exposed to rabies can give birth to kittens that are carrying the virus. Rabies is a very serious disease, one that can cause fatalities in humans as well as in cats and other mammals. For this reason, it cannot be recommended that you hand-raise kittens that could have come from an exposed queen. Kittens should be euthanized if they are found abandoned in areas where rabies is common. If you are in doubt, contact your local health department about the prevalence of rabies in your area.

If Your Kittens Get Sick

With luck, your orphans will thrive on the formula and care that you provide. However, everything does not always go as planned. Your kittens may develop problems that you should be prepared to solve.

Failure to Nurse

Refusing to eat is not a disease—it is a sign of something serious going wrong. A healthy, young animal eagerly consumes enough food to sustain its life and growth.

Kittens that fail to nurse from the beginning are often suffering from damage caused by chilling and starvation. Previous chapters include information about warming and feeding newborn kittens. Remember to give them readily available fluid and calories. Your veterinarian can help if the fluid must be administered by injection.

Diarrhea

Loose, watery stools often come before other signs of illness. Sudden failure to nurse is often a sequel to diarrhea. Usually, diarrhea occurs for a day or two before the kittens become weak, dehydrated, and stop nursing.

Kittens' stools should be soft, yellowish, and definitely formed. If the stools are mushy or watery, immediately dilute the kittens' milk formula with one-third volume plain water. If their diarrhea is not relieved, dilute the formula with one-half plain water. Give the same amount of the diluted formula as you did the regular formula.

When the kittens' stools become formed, gradually return to the full-strength formula over a period of 24 hours. If your kittens do not make a speedy recovery, consult your veterinarian. Perhaps the kittens need to receive oral antibiotics. Perhaps your kittens cannot digest the formula.

If your kittens become too weak to nurse from a bottle, you may have to feed them with a tube. When the kittens are stronger, you can once again feed them with the bottle.

Eye Problems

Kittens' eyes normally open between their fifth and fourteenth day of life. This large difference results from the normal variation of kittens' development at birth. Kittens' eyes are more likely to open at five days than at ten or more days. If kittens' lids are not parted at fourteen days, something is probably wrong.

Check your kittens' eyes daily. If swelling appears behind the unopened lids of kittens of any age, the kittens may have a bacterial eye infection. The kittens' eyes will be damaged permanently unless you take action.

How can you tell if your kittens have this problem? Their closed lids will bulge out from their sockets. The eye areas of each of the kittens may not be the same; some will be swollen and some will not. If you are unsure, ask your veterinarian to examine the kittens.

The treatment for infections of kittens' unopened eyes is twofold. First, the kittens' eyelids must be parted to allow the removal of purulent material. This is usually a job for a veterinarian. Second, you must place antibiotic ointment into the opened eyes at least every eight hours for a minimum of seven days or until the infection is completely eliminated.

You must prevent your kittens' eyelids from becoming stuck together. Wash each kitten's eyes with a cotton ball dipped into warm water before you apply the eye ointment. If a kitten has only one affected eye, its other eye will soon become affected. Open and treat both eyes at the same time. Examine all the kittens. Seemingly unaffected kittens in the litter (even if you house them in separate boxes) may develop the same infection.

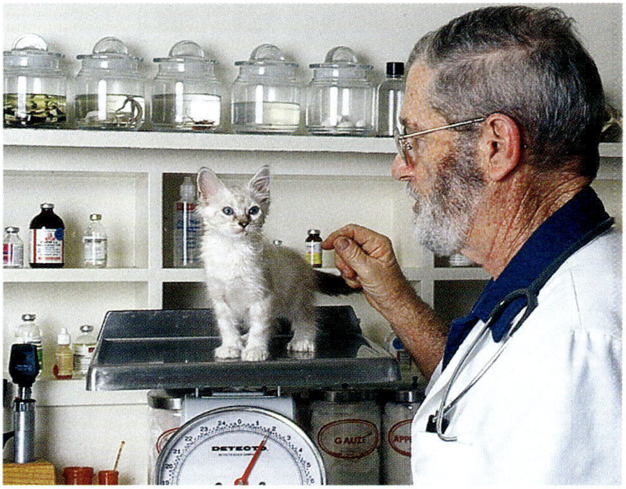

The veterinarian will weigh your kitten to check its growth.

Eye infections commonly occur in older kittens. Kittens whose eyes have opened naturally may develop stuck-together lids. Clean these kittens' eyes, and treat them with antibiotic ointment.

1. Wash all the exudate off each kitten's eyes with a cotton ball and warm water. Use a new cotton ball for each kitten.

2. Apply antibiotic ointment (prescribed or dispensed by your veterinarian) to each cleaned eye at least every eight hours.

3. Continue this treatment for at least five days or until the kittens' eyes have been completely free of discharge for three or more days.

Fading Kitten Syndrome

Kittens occasionally become weak, stop nursing, and die in spite of the most conscientious and dedicated attention. Often, the cause of these deaths can be determined only by a complete autopsy that must include microscopic examination of the dead kittens' tissues and bacterial cultures of their intestinal contents.

If kittens fade and die soon after birth, they likely suffered irreversible damage from hypoglycemia and low body temperatures before you tried to save them. Kittens that die unexpectedly at two weeks or older may have hidden abnormalities that prevent them from thriving. If you attempt to hand-raise kittens, do not be discouraged if some of them do not make it. Nobody can raise them all.

Protecting Your Kittens' Health

If your kittens never received colostrum from their birth mother, they will have less immunity to disease than kittens that nursed normally for the first day of their lives. Isolating colostrum-deprived kittens from possible sources of infection such as other cats and environmental contaminants is wise.

Fecal Examination

By the time your kittens are three weeks old, every litter should have a fecal sample examined under a microscope by a veterinarian or a veterinary technician. A sample that contains fecal matter from two or more littermates is sufficient to detect parasites in the intestines of the entire litter. If the three-week sample is negative, the veterinarian or technician should reexamine samples from the litter at two-week intervals until the kittens are at least nine weeks old. If any sample is positive, the kittens should be treated and rechecked as indicated by your veterinarian.

Vaccinating Your Kittens

Many virus diseases affect only cats and closely related animals. Among these diseases are feline distemper or *panleukopenia;* feline respiratory diseases such as *rhinotracheitis, calicivirus,* and *chalmydia;* and feline leukemia. Some of these diseases are common only in certain areas in the nation, while some diseases are prevalent everywhere. Rely on your veterinarian to make recommendations appropriate to your kittens' circumstances.

Queen-raised kittens usually begin to receive vaccinations when they are seven or eight weeks of age. Hand-raised kittens that did not receive colostrum often start receiving vaccinations at five or six weeks of age.

Rabies vaccine should be administered to all kittens over three months of age. A rabies booster vaccine should be given when the kittens are a year old. Additional rabies booster vaccines should be

given according to the recommendations of your veterinarian.

Neutering Your Kittens

Prepubertal neutering—the spaying or castration of kittens before they reach the age of puberty—was first promoted by humane societies. Cute little kittens are considered more adoptable than are older cats. However, allowing the adoption of unaltered kittens presents the risk that their new owners will fail to have the surgery done. Prepubertal neutering was the answer. Small kittens can be adopted after they have been surgically sterilized.

Recently, the American Veterinary Medical Association has examined the practice of prepubertal sterilization. The association has reached the following conclusions:

- The surgery is *not* more difficult to perform than is surgery on mature animals.
- Young animals are *not* more difficult to anesthetize than are older ones. Nor is there more risk from anesthesia to prepubertal animals than to mature animals.
- Young animals recover from anesthesia and surgery more rapidly than do older ones.
- Early altering eliminates the risk that the animal will reach puberty sooner than expected. Unexpected pregnancies and undesirable sexual behavior are eliminated. Urine spraying in the house is curtailed.
- Studies indicate that early neutering has no undesirable side effects. Research has been proven that early castration does not change cats' urinary tracts.
- Neutered kittens can be adopted with no risk that they will reproduce. Humane societies are concerned with population control. They all advocate prepubertal altering for this reason alone.

Should you have your kittens surgically sterilized before they reach puberty? If you plan to keep the kittens, the answer is yes. You will save yourself the trouble of your female kitten coming into heat before you realize she has. You will prevent your male kitten from spraying in the house before you realize that he has become sexually mature.

If you are planning to find new homes for your hand-raised orphans, you may prefer that their new owners incur the expense of the surgery. Be sure your kittens go only to people who will not allow the kittens to reproduce. Far too many kittens in the world are homeless now.

A few veterinarians still insist that kittens be six months or older to spay, nine months or older to castrate. This practice is not harmful if you are lucky enough to have the surgery done before your kittens reach sexual maturity.

Chapter Ten

Parasitic Infections

Many kittens die from the harm that parasites do to their bodies. Parasites invade kittens' organs, suck their blood, consume their nutrients, and block their intestines. You need not allow this to happen. In the majority of instances, informed owners can recognize and deal with parasites before their kittens have suffered irreparable damage.

A *parasite* is an organism that must spend part or all of its life living on or within the body of another organism. The plant or animal upon which a parasite lives is called the *host.*

All parasites are harmful. Some parasites are so harmful that the survival of their hosts is seriously affected. Some parasites are so innocuous that their hosts can live with them for their entire lives. Cats host a large number of parasites, many of which can be present in newborn kittens. Some parasites in kittens should be eliminated as soon as they are discovered. Some cannot be eliminated until the kittens are large enough and strong enough to withstand treatment. Your kittens certainly will be healthier after their parasites have been eliminated.

Some drugs that are safe for dogs are poisonous to cats. Obtain safe drugs for cats from your veterinarian. Read every word on the label of every drug package.

Internal Parasites

Parasites that live within the body of their hosts, *internal* parasites, are commonly called worms, although some are not the long, thin, classic worm shape. The adult forms of most internal parasites of the cat live in the intestines. Many immature stages of worms migrate through the cat hosts' blood vessels or tissues. Parasites relatively harmless to adult cats may cause serious or even fatal diseases in tiny kittens.

Roundworms

Toxocara sp., the cat roundworm, is a common parasite of kittens. Adult roundworms in cats and kittens are up to 3 inches (8 cm) in length. They are called roundworms

because they are round in cross section, like spaghetti.

Adult roundworms live in the kittens' or cats' small intestine. The immature forms of roundworms migrate throughout the cats' bodies, where they may form cysts in the tissues of affected animals.

Roundworm cysts in the mother's tissues are the source of infection for newborn kittens. Cystic larvae in cats' tissues may be inactive for the entire life of a male or a spayed female cat. When an unspayed female cat that has roundworm cysts in her tissues becomes pregnant, the cysts become active. The larvae are released to become adult roundworms.

When these larvae become adult worms in the intestine of the mother cat, her feces will contain worm eggs that can infect her kittens. If the worm larvae migrate into the cat's mammary glands, the kittens can become infected as they nurse.

Adult roundworms damage kittens' intestinal systems; larval roundworms harm the tissues of the kitten through which they migrate. Diarrhea and poor weight gain are the two most common signs of roundworm infestation in kittens.

Adult roundworms, which are rarely passed in kittens' stools, may be from ½ to 3 inches (1 to 8 cm) long and easily visible. Each adult female roundworm can produce up to 20,000 microscopic eggs a day. Roundworm infections in kittens are diagnosed by microscopic examination of the kittens' stools. Take a

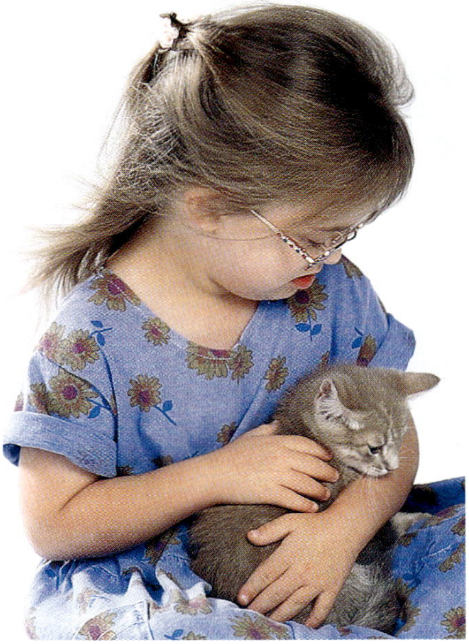

Teach children to wash their hands after they pet the kittens.

sample of your kittens' fecal material to your veterinarian. Include a small amount of feces from several of your kittens. Your veterinarian (or the veterinary technician) will treat the sample with methods that help find worm eggs under the microscope. If the stool sample is negative, the veterinarian will recommend that the kittens' stools be checked several more times to be sure that the kittens are not harboring the parasite.

If your veterinarian finds roundworm eggs in your kittens' stools, he or she will prescribe medication to treat the infection. Your veterinarian will ask you to bring stool samples after the kittens have been treated to be sure the worms have all been eliminated. Several treatments are often required before the

Kittens may be harmed by drugs that are safe for older cats. Always check with your veterinarian before you give any medication!

kittens' intestines are free of roundworms.

Tapeworms

The tapeworm must live in the bodies of two entirely different species of hosts to complete its life cycle. The *intermediate host* harbors the immature stages of tapeworms, the *final host* harbors the adult tapeworms. Different species of immature cat tapeworms live in one of two hosts: mice or fleas. The mouse or flea is the *intermediate host.* Adult forms of the cat tapeworm live in cats or kittens. The cat is the *final host.*

The adult forms of most tapeworms are long and flat, like a ribbon or a piece of tape. Each tapeworm consists of a *scolex* (head) attached to the lining of the host's intestines. A long chain of segments containing tapeworm eggs develops from each scolex. The segments break off the end of the chain and leave the cat's body with its stool.

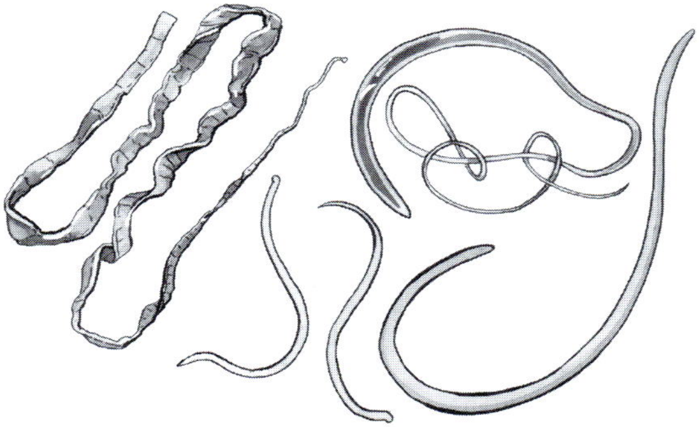

Tapeworm, whipworm, roundworm, and hookworm.

Tapeworm segments can be seen on the surface of the host's stool or crawling from the host's anus. Fresh segments are white and able to wiggle. Old tapeworm segments dry and resemble a grain of rice attached to the hair around the anal area of the cat.

Mice become infected with tapeworms when they feed on tapeworm segments passed by a cat. Flea larvae feed upon debris in the environment, including tapeworm segments. Fleas contain the immature form of tapeworms when flea larvae that have eaten tapeworm segments become adults. A cat (the final host) that eats mice or a cat that licks itself and swallows fleas can become infected with tapeworms.

Newborn kittens, of course, do not eat mice. Kittens that have never eaten mice will not be infected with the species of tapeworm for which the mouse is the intermediate host. When they nurse from a flea-infested mother, newborn kittens can and do get fleas in their mouths and swallow them by accident. If the fleas contain tapeworm larvae, the kittens will become infected with tapeworms.

Seldom can tapeworms be diagnosed by a microscopic examination of kittens' stools because the tapeworm eggs are contained in the segments and are not dispersed in the fecal matter. Look for moving segments on your kittens' anal areas. If the kittens or their mother

have had fleas, you may observe them passing tapeworm segments at a surprisingly young age—sometimes as young as eight weeks. Your veterinarian will prescribe one of the new drugs that eliminate tapeworms and are safe for kittens.

Human tapeworms are spread in some parts of the world when people eat undercooked fish. Humans rarely get cat or dog tapeworms even if they swallow infective fleas or mice.

Hookworms

The dog hookworm occurs occasionally in cats in the United States. Because queens with hookworms may pass the infection to their kittens in their first milk (colostrum), this parasite may be present in very young kittens. Older cats and dogs get this parasite by licking or eating objects contaminated with infective hookworm eggs. Evidence shows that the larval hoookworms may also gain entrance into the body by penetrating the foot pads of cats and dogs, just as the human hookworm penetrates the soles of children's bare feet.

Hookworms cause damage to kittens and puppies by sucking blood from the walls of their hosts' intestines. A very heavy hookworm infection will cause the host to be anemic from chronic blood loss. Thin, poorly growing kittens with dark, smelly, loose stools may be suffering from hookworm. The condition is diagnosed by finding the characteristic eggs in the kittens' stool under a microscope. In the unlikely instance that your kittens have hookworms, your veterinarian or veterinary technician will find it at the same time he or she looks for roundworm eggs. Some medications that eliminate roundworms also act against hookworms.

Coccidia

Coccidia belong to a group of one-celled organisms known as *protozoa.* Coccidiosis (an infection with coccidia) commonly occurs in kittens. A heavy infection of coccidia can damage a kitten's small intestine enough to cause blood loss, severe diarrhea, dehydration, and death.

Newborn kittens occasionally get coccidiosis from ingesting coccidia oocysts on the fur of their mothers. Older kittens get coccidiosis by licking their paws contaminated with feces from other infected animals. If your kittens have coccidiosis, the characteristic oocysts of coccidia will be found when their stools are examined under the microscope.

Coccidiosis is dangerous to kittens when the organisms are present in great numbers in the kittens' intestines. If treated early, these parasites can be eliminated before doing serious harm to your kittens. This condition is treated with a sulfonamide drug prescribed by your veterinarian.

No drug controls every species of parasite. If your kittens have more than one parasite, they may need more than one drug.

Toxoplasma

Toxoplasma gondii is a one-celled parasite of cats, similar to coccidia. An infection with *T. gondii* is called *toxoplasmosis.*

Felines are the *definitive,* or *final, hosts* of *T. gondii*. Many animals can be the *intermediate* host of this parasite, including rodents, birds, dogs, hoofed animals, and humans.

The larvae of *T. gondii* in the tissues of infected female animals can migrate through the placenta into the fetuses. The larvae can migrate into mothers' mammary glands and be present in the milk. Kittens born to queens with toxoplasmosis may become infected with this parasite before they are born and when they nurse.

Adult cats infected with toxoplasma often are carriers of the parasite, but are not sick. Kittens and young cats are more likely to have signs of the disease, such as pneumonia, fever, and bloody diarrhea. Making a positive diagnosis of toxoplasmosis in cats and kittens is difficult. The oocysts of this parasite are very small and are passed in the feces of infected cats for only a limited time. Infected kittens may not pass oocysts for weeks or months.

Adult cats acquire toxoplasma from eating infected intermediate hosts (mice, birds) or from eating undercooked meat from infected animals. For this reason, you can best prevent your cats from contracting toxoplasmosis by keeping them indoors where they cannot catch and eat rodents or birds and by never feeding them undercooked meat.

Toxoplasmosis and roundworms may be a threat to humans. Chapter 11 explains the hazards of these parasites.

Heartworm

Adult heartworms live in the chambers of the heart and the major blood vessels of the host. Heartworms do not lay eggs. Instead, they produce hundreds of microscopic larvae called *microfilaria.* Microfilaria circulate in the blood of the host.

Mosquitoes act as the intermediate hosts of this deadly parasite. When a mosquito feeds on a heartworm-infected animal, it sucks up the microfilaria with the animal's blood. The mosquito can then transmit the microfilaria to other animals upon which it feeds.

Dirofilaria immitis is the heartworm that infects cats as well as dogs. Signs of the infection in cats are not the same as signs of infection in dogs. Dogs may live with many heartworms for years before they gradually develop signs of breathing difficulties and circulatory disturbance. Dogs with subclinical heartworm infection can usually be treated and cured of the condition. Cats with the disease often have only one or two heartworms in their circulatory systems. Affected cats may die suddenly without previous signs of illness. Treating cats with heartworms carries a much greater risk than treat-

ing dogs with heartworms. Veterinarians often prefer not to risk the death of infected cats by treating them for this parasitic disease.

You need not worry about heartworm in hand-raised kittens until they are weaned. Although very young kittens may have been bitten by mosquitoes, the life cycle of the heartworm is such that preventive treatment can start when kittens are four months old. Your veterinarian will recommend a monthly dose of preventive medication for your kittens. Tell the owners of the kittens you place into new homes to ask their veterinarians about this essential protection.

External Parasites

External parasites are creatures that live on the skin or within the layers of the skin of the host. Some external parasites spend their entire lives on the same host. Other external parasites inhabit the skin of the host only during certain stages of their lives. Some external parasites must live on two or more different host species in order to complete their life cycles.

Some external parasites are extremely *species specific* and can live on only one species of host. Other parasites are not species specific and can use many kinds of animals as their hosts. Many external parasites prefer a specific host but will infest other hosts if their preferred host is not present.

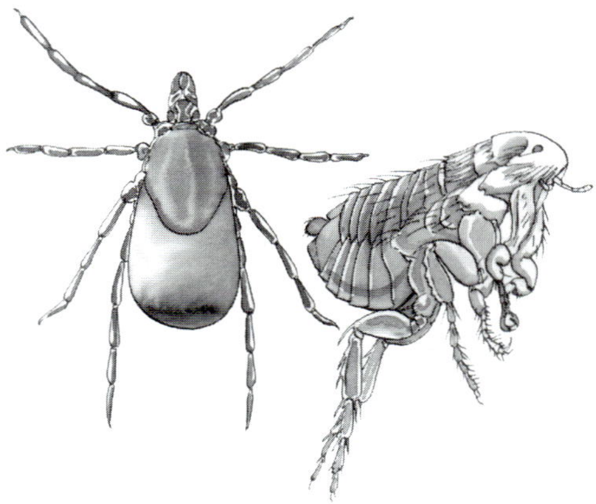

A tick and a flea.

The adults of most external parasites are multicellular animals visible to the naked eye. The eggs of these parasites are often too small to be seen without a microscope or a magnifying lens. Some external parasites are visible on newborn kittens; some will become apparent only when the kittens grow.

Fleas

Almost everyone can identify fleas. These small, dark insects run through their host's fur and can jump several inches to inhabit new hosts. Abandoned newborn kittens have seldom had good care. Often, they are covered with fleas.

Adult fleas live on the host animal. The adults lay microscopic flea eggs on the host that then fall off into the host's bedding. The eggs hatch into larvae that resemble tiny, hairy caterpillars. These larvae eat debris, including tapeworm segments and the fecal material of adult fleas that drop off the host. A flea larva molts several times before

Only a veterinarian with a microscope can be sure that this kitten is free of parasites.

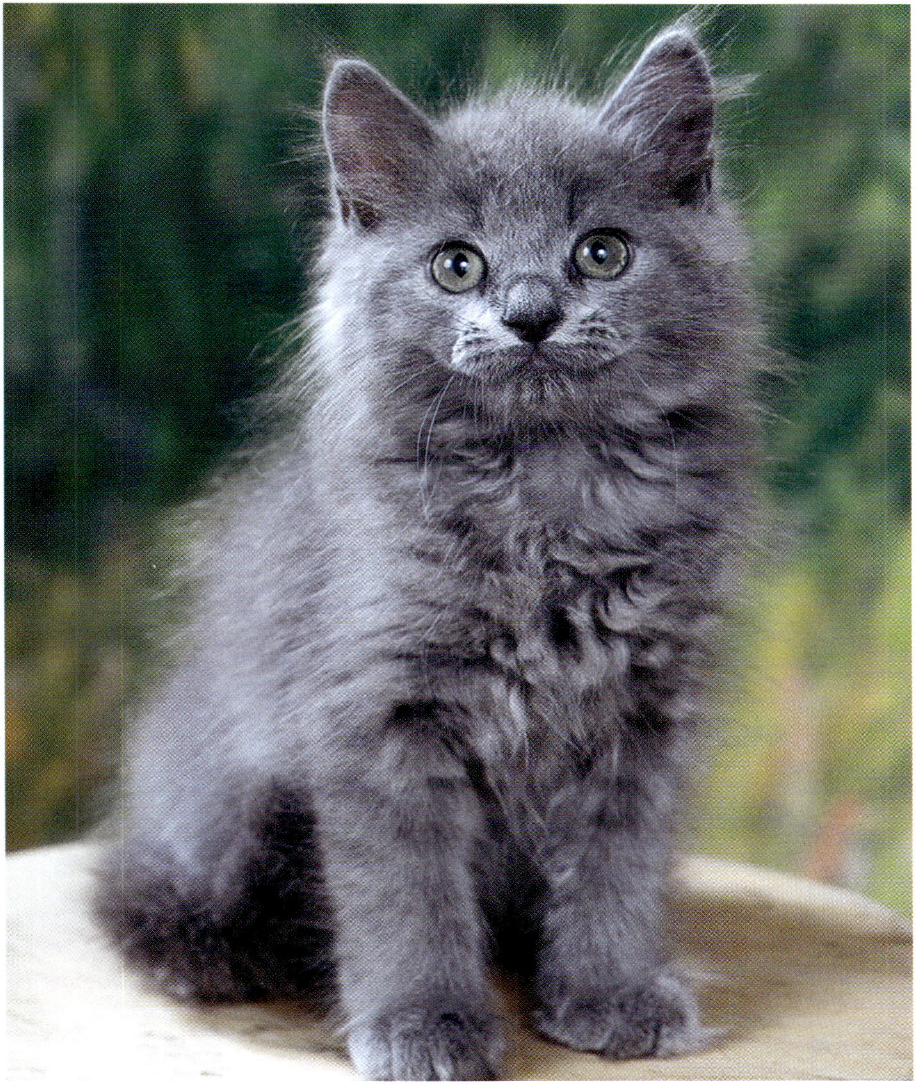

it forms a pupa (cocoon). Eventually, the flea emerges from its pupa as an adult in search of a host. The fleas on your newborn kittens crawled onto them from the queen or jumped onto them from the nest

In cats and older kittens, fleas cause a great deal of scratching and resultant skin abrasion. When accidentally swallowed, fleas can transmit tapeworm infection to kittens and cats. However, the major

damage done to tiny kittens by fleas is from blood loss.

Adult fleas are blood-sucking parasites. The black, gritty *flea dirt* on your flea-infested kittens is flea feces, composed mainly of partly digested blood. Prove this to yourself. Scrape a bit of flea dirt onto a piece of white paper and add a drop of water. The paper will turn reddish brown from the red blood cells in the flea droppings. Kittens that harbor a large number of fleas can become anemic, weak, and even die from the constant loss of blood caused by fleas.

Eliminating fleas from newborn kittens is extremely important. If you find that your kittens are infested, attack the problem from two directions.

First remove the fleas from your kittens. Flea powders and shampoos may contain chemicals that will harm kittens under a month of age. Removing the fleas without using insecticides may be best. Comb fleas off your kittens with a fine-toothed comb from a drugstore or a *flea comb* from a pet store. First rub mineral oil onto the teeth of the comb to trap the fleas. Then run the comb through the kittens' fur. Finally, rinse the comb in soapy water to drown the fleas as you capture them. In extreme cases, you may have to swish your kittens in a basin of warm water to drown and float the fleas from their coats. Be careful to keep the kittens' heads above water and to dry them thoroughly. Before you use any insecticides, check with your veterinarian to be sure the product is safe.

The second step is eliminating flea eggs, larvae, and pupae from your kittens' beds. This step is essential to prevent your kittens from getting new fleas. Take all the bedding, including newspapers, towels, and blankets, out of your kittens' boxes. If possible, discard cardboard boxes and get new ones. If you do not have new boxes, carefully clean the cracks of the old boxes with a vacuum tool before you put in new papers and bedding. Burn the old papers, or throw them away where hatching fleas cannot jump onto your kittens. If you want to use the towels again, wash them in your washer with laundry soap and hot water, then dry them in a clothes drier set on hot or dry. Hot water and soap and the heat of the dryer will kill immature stages of fleas. If your heating pads have cloth covers, do not forget to wash and dry these also.

Mites

Adult mites are microscopic or almost microscopic. They spend their entire lives on the body of the host and are spread when an infected animal comes into contact with an uninfected one. If your kittens' mother had mites, your newborn kittens may possibly have mites also.

Ear mites, *Otodectes cynotis,* commonly infest cats and kittens. In adult cats and older kittens, these mites cause their hosts to scratch their ears

and shake their heads. The ears of infected cats and kittens contain a crusty, thick, brown-black wax in which the mites live and reproduce.

Kittens' ear canals are closed at birth and do not open until the kittens are from 5 to 12 days old. Kittens acquire ear mites from their mothers only after their ear canals are open and before they are weaned. However, if your kittens' mother had ear mites, some of the mites may live on the kittens' skin until they can infect the kittens' ear canals. Your kittens' ear canals will open at or about the same time their eyes open. Check your kittens' ears often. If you see crusty, black material, ask your veterinarian how to treat the condition.

Another mite that affects cats, *Notoedres cati,* occurs much less commonly than the ear mite. This parasite lives on the head and neck of cats and kittens. It may spread to the hosts' entire body and causes intense scratching and scabbing. If your kittens' mother had this mite, your kittens will be infected. Kittens' infection will not be apparent until the kittens are old enough to scratch themselves.

Notoedres mites are microscopic in size. They occur plentifully on infected kittens and cats. Veterinarians and veterinary technicians can easily find them by examining a skin scraping under the microscope. If your kittens scratch or have skin lesions, ask your veterinarian to check for these mites.

Both *Otodectes* and *Notoedres* mites are easily treated with modern drugs. Oral or topical medication will kill *Otodectes* ear mites. Oral medication given as soon as the affected kittens are old enough to eat solid food will eliminate *Notoedres* mites. These mites are extremely contagious to other cats. If other cats have had contact with infected kittens, the cats should be treated as a precaution.

Both cat and dog mites can cause mild, transient skin rashes on the hands and arms of humans. These mites are not the same as the human scabies mite; they will not live long on people. The rash on humans caused by cat mites goes away without treatment within a day or two.

Ticks

Ticks rarely occur on kittens. Since many hand-raised kittens come from unknown sources, some may have been born in wooded, tick-infested areas. These kittens occasionally have adult or immature ticks attached to their skin.

Ticks must live on at least two host animals to complete their life cycles. They are opportunistic when selecting their hosts. Most ticks will live on many species of wild rodents, carnivores, and animals with hooves. In between the times they are living on a host, ticks develop on the ground or elsewhere in the environment.

Male and unfed female ticks resemble small, fat spiders that are relatively stationary on their hosts. Immature ticks can be very tiny and easy to overlook; adult ticks are large enough to be visible. When

ticks become engorged with blood, they resemble dark, round masses of ¼ to ½ inch (6 to 13 mm) in length. You can most commonly find ticks in the ears and between the toes of an affected animal.

Ticks can carry several diseases that can be transmitted to other animals including humans. These diseases include Rocky Mountain spotted fever, tick paralysis, and Lyme disease. If you find even one tick, check each kitten every day. Ticks that are too small to be found will grow enough in only one or two days to be detected easily.

Ticks are hard to kill. Insecticides that kill ticks will also harm your newborn kittens. You must remove ticks on kittens by hand. If you find anything that might be a tick, pull it off your kitten with tweezers. If you yank a tick off with your fingers, use rubber gloves or several layers of tissue to protect your hands. Do not handle a tick with your bare hands.

If your kittens are two weeks or more of age, you can kill ticks before you remove them. Apply tick spray to a cotton ball and hold the ball against the tick. After a minute of this treatment, the tick will be dead or dying when you pull it off.

Drop the tick into a jar, screw the lid on tightly, and take it to your veterinarian for identification. Wipe alcohol on any kitten's skin where the tick was attached. Do not worry that the mouthparts of the tick may remain in the kitten's skin. If this happens, the mouthparts will soon dry up and drop off the kitten's skin.

If you find ticks on your kittens, throw away their cardboard boxes and all their bedding. Ticks have been known to live on clothing through the entire wash and dry cycle of a home laundry.

Lice

Lice are extremely *host specific.* Many animals, including humans, may have lice. However, each species of louse lives on only one species of animal. Human lice will not live on cats, cat lice will not live on humans. If your children come home with head lice, they did not get them from your kittens. They got human lice from their friends at school.

A kitten infected with lice will have scabby dandruff and greasy-looking skin. If you suspect that your kittens have lice, pick up some of the scales and dandruff by using the sticky side of a piece of Scotch tape. Examine the tape in a strong light with a magnifying lens. Small, soft, white insects stuck to the tape are lice. Tiny white beads attached to the hair shafts are the nits, or eggs, of the louse.

Lice spend their entire lives on a single animal. They can live only a few hours off a host. Lice are transmitted to other animals by close contact, such as by a mother cat to her kittens. Lice are easy to kill with mild insecticides, but the nits are resistant. You must repeat the treatment every few days until all the nits have hatched and been eliminated. Your veterinarian will prescribe a

Children can get ringworm from infected kittens; have your kitten examined by a veterinarian.

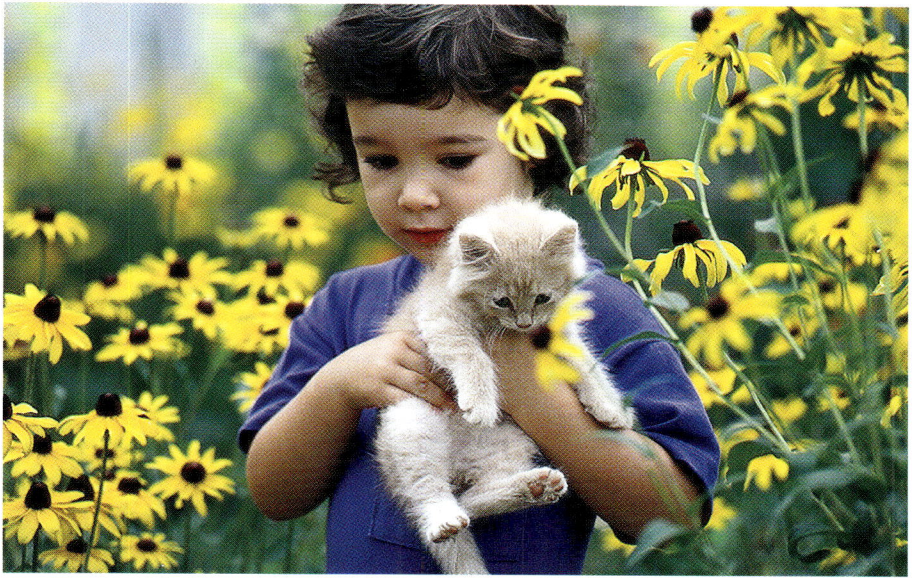

product that will kill lice but is harmless to kittens.

Ringworm

A microscopic fungus causes ringworm. *Microsporum canis* is the common organism that causes ringworm in cats and dogs. This organism can also infect other animals, including humans. Many adult cats are carriers of ringworm but have no signs of the disease. Infected queens, even if they have no signs of ringworm, spread it to their kittens. Kittens and children are much more likely to have skin lesions from ringworm than are cats and adult humans.

The name ringworm comes from the growth pattern of the organism. The organism grows outward from the initial site of infection, forming circles or rings of hairless, scaly, inflamed areas. On kittens, these lesions most commonly appear on the face, ears, and paws.

Infected kittens will seldom have visible ringworm lesions until they are two or three months old. Children like to handle kittens. Children can get ringworm from infected kittens even before the kittens have ringworm lesions themselves. Asking your veterinarian to examine your kittens under a Wood's light as a precautionary measure is wise even if they have no sign of the disease.

A vaccine against ringworm is now available for cats. Although the vaccine is intended to prevent ringworm, it also produces significant improvement in kittens that already have the disease. Your veterinarian can tell you if and when your kittens should receive this vaccine.

Chapter Eleven

Zoonoses: Diseases Shared by Cats and Humans

A *zoonosis* is a disease that animals and humans can share. Nothing in life is entirely without risk. Certain disease organisms can spread from cats to humans and occasionally from humans to cats. As an informed owner, you can take the necessary steps to minimize the problem of diseases that you and your family can share with your kittens.

Some zoonoses occur very rarely, some are uncommon, and some occur with great frequency. Some zoonoses are serious or even fatal to affected animals and humans; some diseases do not cause much harm. Some diseases are hard to cure, some are readily treated with modern drugs. A few zoonoses affect only humans and cats. Most that affect humans and cats are also capable of infecting dogs and other animals.

Avoiding contact with cats or kittens because humans and felines can share certain diseases is not necessary. However, you must take appropriate precautions to protect yourself, your family, and your cats.

Rabies

Rabies is a deadly disease that affects wild and domestic mammals, including humans. It is a contagious viral disease that almost always results in fatality in infected animals. The rabies virus attacks the nervous system. Signs of rabies infection include abnormal behavior, increased excitability, and eventual paralysis.

The virus reproduces in the salivary glands of rabid animals. Rabies is transmitted to other animals when the saliva of an infected

The diseases described are some of the more common zoonoses. If you suspect other problems, consult your veterinarian immediately.

Kittens and children like to get close. Take precautions to minimize problems with diseases shared by cats and humans.

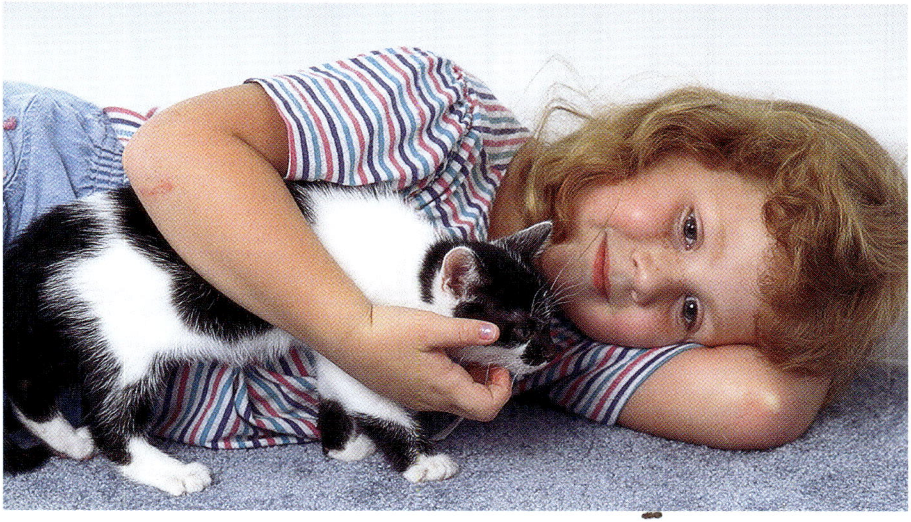

animal enters a bite wound or the broken skin of an uninfected animal. Raccoons, skunks, foxes, bats, and coyotes are the most common reservoirs of rabies virus.

Every species of mammal can become infected with the rabies virus, although some species are more resistant than others to the disease. Among the more resistant species are humans and opossums; among the more susceptible species are cattle and foxes. Rabies has seldom been found in wild rodents, perhaps because rodents rarely survive the bite of a rabid predator. Rabies spreads to human handlers when pet animals or cattle are infected by rabid wildlife.

A rabid animal can spread rabies to other animals during only the few days that the rabies virus appears in its saliva. Unfortunately, the incubation period of rabies varies. Many factors influence the length of time between infection and the onset of disease.

Incubation periods of between 9 and 60 days have been reported in cats. Veterinarians do not know if a cat infected with rabies can complete a pregnancy and deliver live kittens while rabies is developing in the queen's body. They do not know if kittens delivered by an infected cat can harbor the rabies virus or can become infected with the virus from their mother.

These two procedures can almost entirely prevent rabies in humans:

1. All domestic mammals must be vaccinated.

2. All contact with possibly rabid wild animals must be avoided.

When someone finds kittens abandoned in the wild, they know nothing about the kittens' mother. The mother cat may have wandered away; she may have been killed by a car; she may have died of a disease. Since so many facts about rabies are unknown, and since rabies is so deadly a disease, the following recommendation must be reluctantly made: Motherless kittens found abandoned in the wild should be euthanized.

Kittens should be hand-raised only if they have no chance of posing a serious threat to the health of their benefactors. Rabies is not a disease with which to take chances.

Ringworm

As discussed in Chapter 10, ringworm is a common skin fungus of cats. Adult cats may be carriers of the disease without having any evidence on their skin. Kittens catch ringworm from their mothers while they nurse. However, infected kittens may be several weeks of age before the disease becomes apparent.

Microsporum canis, the organism that causes the majority of ringworm on cats, is readily spread by contact to dogs and children. Veterinarians diagnose ringworm in kittens by using one or more of these methods:

1. Examination of the animal under a Wood's light. This device emits ultraviolet rays. If ringworm fungus is present, it may appear to fluoresce.

2. Microscopic examination of hairs plucked from infected areas and treated with chemicals. Veterinarians or veterinary technicians may see fungus spores along the shafts of infected hairs.

3. A culture made from suspected hairs on a substance that promotes fungus growth. If fungus is present, it will be identifiable within seven to ten days.

None of these diagnostic methods is infallible. False negative findings commonly occur.

Even if your kittens' skin appears to be completely normal, ask your veterinarian to perform a Wood's light examination of your kittens. If you have reason to suspect ringworm, such as hairless patches on your kittens' heads or front paws, request that your veterinarian perform the other tests as well.

Treatment of newborn kittens for ringworm usually must wait until the kittens are older. Your veterinarian will prescribe topical or oral medication when your kittens are two to three months of age.

Adult humans seem to be relatively resistant to the ringworm organism, but the infection readily spreads to children. If any of the tests indicate that your kittens are positive, do not allow children to handle the kittens.

The ringworm organism can be spread not only from kitten to child but from child to child and from child to kitten. Your child may get ringworm from a schoolmate and infect your kittens. If you suspect ringworm in your children, consult your pediatrician or dermatologist.

Nursing kittens will ingest roundworm larvae in their mother's milk.

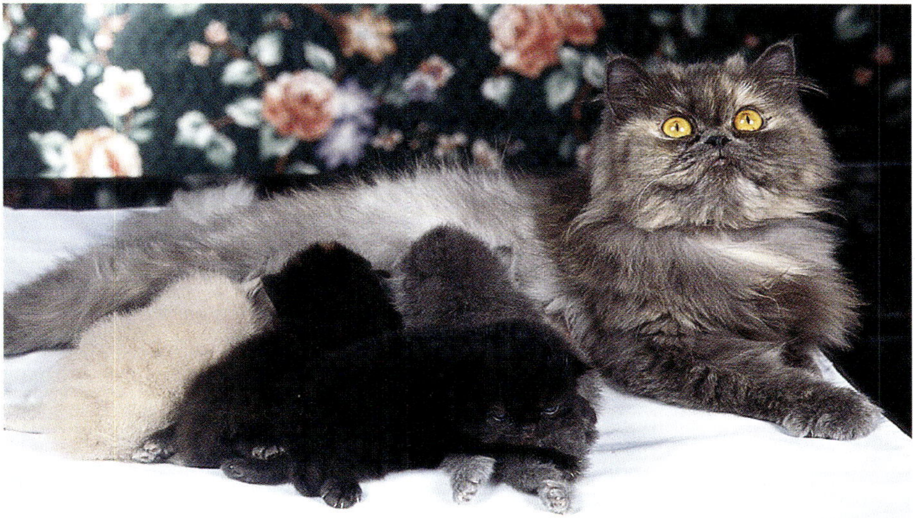

Cat Roundworms

The common cat roundworm, *Toxocara cati,* can complete its life cycle in only domestic and wild members of the cat family. Kittens become infected with this parasite in one of two ways:

1. As nursing kittens, they ingest roundworm larvae in their mother's milk.

2. As weaned kittens, they swallow infective eggs or larvae passed in the feces of their mother or other cats.

Roundworm larvae migrate from the kittens' stomachs and enter their tissues. The larvae then migrate through the kittens' lungs and become adult roundworms in the kittens' intestines. These adult roundworms produce thousands of eggs that are passed in the kittens' stools.

Children who play in areas contaminated with cat feces or who handle kittens infected with roundworms can get the microscopic eggs of this parasite on their hands. If they put their hands into their mouths, children can accidentally swallow roundworm eggs.

When a human swallows infective *T. cati* eggs, the eggs hatch into larvae in the human's stomach, just as they hatched into larvae in the kittens' stomachs. These larvae can migrate through human tissues. However, they cannot complete their life cycle in humans. Cat roundworms cannot become adult worms in human intestines.

Humans, most often children, suffer damage from cat roundworm larvae migrating through their tissues. *Toxocaral larva migrans* is the condition in which the roundworm lar-

vae damage an infected human's internal organs, eyes, and brain.

Both the cat roundworm, *T. cati,* and the dog roundworm, *T. canis,* can cause human cases of toxocaral larva migrans. Infection of humans from puppies and dogs occurs much more commonly than infection of humans from kittens. You can minimize the slight risk present when you handle kittens by following a few simple precautions.

- Wash your hands! Wash with soap and hot, running water each time you handle your kittens. Be sure that your children have scrubbed their hands after they touch the kittens.
- Keep the kittens' beds clean. Change their bedding whenever it is soiled. Dispose of the soiled bedding where no other animals can touch it. If you use folded towels for bedding, wash them with soap in the hot cycle of the washer.
- Wash your kittens if their coats become soiled with their feces. Use plain warm water or human baby shampoo to remove all traces of fecal matter from your kittens' fur. Dry the kittens with soft towels, and keep them warm after their baths.
- Treat your kittens with vermifuges for roundworms as soon as your veterinarian tells you they are old enough. Your veterinarian will prescribe appropriate medication. Repeat the treatments at two- to four-week intervals until the kittens are at least three months old.

Wash your hands after handling kittens! Then wash your hands again!

Treat the kittens even if their stool samples are negative for roundworms. All roundworm infections do not show up in every stool sample.

Toxoplasmosis

The definitive host of *Toxoplasma gondii* is the cat. The intermediate hosts of this parasite include many animals such as rodents, dogs, foxes, swine, sheep, cattle, chickens, and humans.

T. gondii has a complicated life cycle. Infection occurs when an animal ingests the oocysts (eggs) passed in the stools of an infected cat or ingests the infective stages of this parasite encysted in the tissues of an intermediate host. Signs of toxoplasmosis in both adult humans and cats are usually mild but can be life threatening. This parasite is probably common but infrequently recognized as the cause of disease in adult animals.

The most serious danger to people from *T. gondii* is congenital toxoplasmosis passed to the unborn fetus from an infected mother. Birth defects that can result from the infection include blindness, brain damage, and stillbirths.

Damage to unborn babies of mothers infected with *T. gondii* is

Pregnant women should not hand-raise kittens!

not common. Do not panic and eliminate cats from the family. Nevertheless, take appropriate precautions to prevent all humans from being infected with toxoplasma. Public health officials recommend the following procedures:

- Since food animals can be the intermediate hosts of this parasite, eat only thoroughly cooked meat. Wash hands after handling raw meat.
- Rodents can be the intermediate hosts of toxoplasma. Keep cats indoors where they cannot hunt and eat rodents. Never feed cats raw or partially cooked meat that might contain infective stages of the parasite.
- Avoid contact with cat feces. Wear gloves when you change litter boxes. Clean and scald litter boxes daily. Dispose of cat feces and used litter in such a way as to prevent contamination of the environment.
- If you are pregnant, do not handle cat feces, even with rubber gloves. Have someone else clean the litter boxes.

Current knowledge about the life cycle of *T. gondii* indicates that this parasite is probably not transmitted from an infected queen to her kittens through the placenta. Kittens are unlikely to become infected with toxoplasma until they are old enough to eat mice. However, it is remotely conceivable that kittens that have recently been in contact with infected queens may be contaminated with the oocysts of toxoplasma.

Hand-raising orphaned kittens always involves some contact with kittens' fecal material. Nursing kittens' feces are very unlikely to contain toxoplasma oocysts. However, obstetricians will be horrified if pregnant women undertake the hand-raising of kittens.

Listen to your doctor. If you are pregnant, do not hand-raise kittens even if you must allow the kittens to be euthanized. Try to find someone else to take over the job.

If you are not pregnant, use the same precautions as you did to prevent infection with roundworm larvae. Wash your hands. Keep the kittens' bedding clean. Be sure your children wash their hands, too.

Cat Scratch Disease

The bacterium *Bartonella henselae* causes cat scratch disease, also called cat scratch fever. Cats can carry this bacterium but seldom get sick from it.

The bacterium gains entrance to the human body from the bite or scratch of an infected cat. Human symptoms include fever, localized rash, and enlarged lymph nodes. Cat scratch disease does not commonly occur and is seldom serious.

With nearly 60 million pet cats in the United States, only about 22,000 cases of cat scratch disease are reported annually.

Researchers at the University of California-Davis have shown that the bacterium that causes cat scratch disease is spread from cat to cat by fleas. If your newborn kittens came to you with fleas, they may have the disease-causing organism in their bodies. Cat scratch disease is not a serious problem when hand-raising orphaned kittens, but take simple precautions to protect yourself:

- Wash your hands every time you handle your kittens.
- Remove fleas from your kittens. Eliminate flea eggs and larvae that will hatch into new fleas and reinfect the kittens.
- Trim the sharp points from your kittens' nails. Give them a soft cloth to cling to instead of your hands.
- If you are even slightly scratched, immediately clean the wound with a disinfectant or wipe it with isopropyl alcohol. Cat scratch disease does not commonly occur, but why take chances?

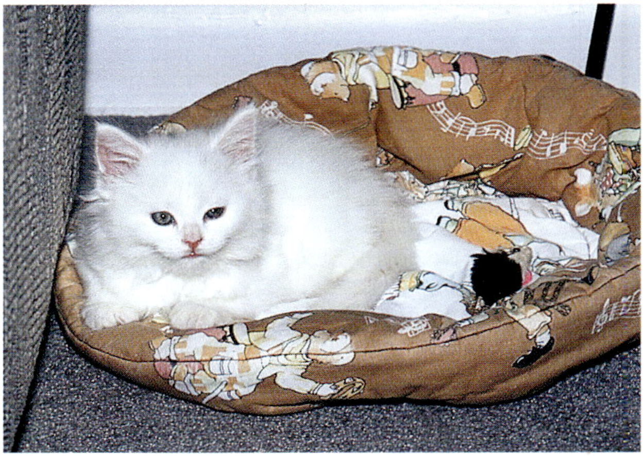

Be sure to keep your kitten's bedding clean.

Chapter Twelve

Feline Overpopulation and Feral Cats

Sixty million cats in the United States have human owners. Unfortunately, another 60 million cats in the United States have no owners at all. Almost nine million cats a year are euthanized in animal shelters.

How did this happen? As many cats are throwaways as are owned in this country. Where did all these cats come from?

Cat Reproduction

A female cat can become pregnant when she is as young as five months of age. She will bear three to six kittens in each litter. Female cats can have two, occasionally three, litters every year. Since half of the kittens are females and since these kittens can get pregnant when they are five months old, the results are obvious: a population explosion.

Enough people do not exist to own all these kittens. Those kittens that nobody wants meet a harsh fate.

- Unwanted cats are discarded at animal control facilities or humane societies. Most of them constitute the nine million cats and kittens euthanized every year. Only a lucky few are placed into new homes.
- Unwanted cats are allowed to wander off the owners' property to "take care of themselves." These cats starve, die from disease or accidents, or reproduce more unwanted kittens.
- Unwanted cats are abandoned far from home. To their "owner," out of sight is out of mind. Abandoned cats meet the same fate as those that wander away. They starve, freeze, die of disease, or are killed by cars or other animals. Those that manage to stay alive become *feral,* the term for a domestic animal gone wild. Sixty million feral cats struggle for existence every day.

Feral cats are scavengers, subsisting on garbage, roadkill, and small rodents. Because garbage is their main source of food, feral cats tend to hang around human habita-

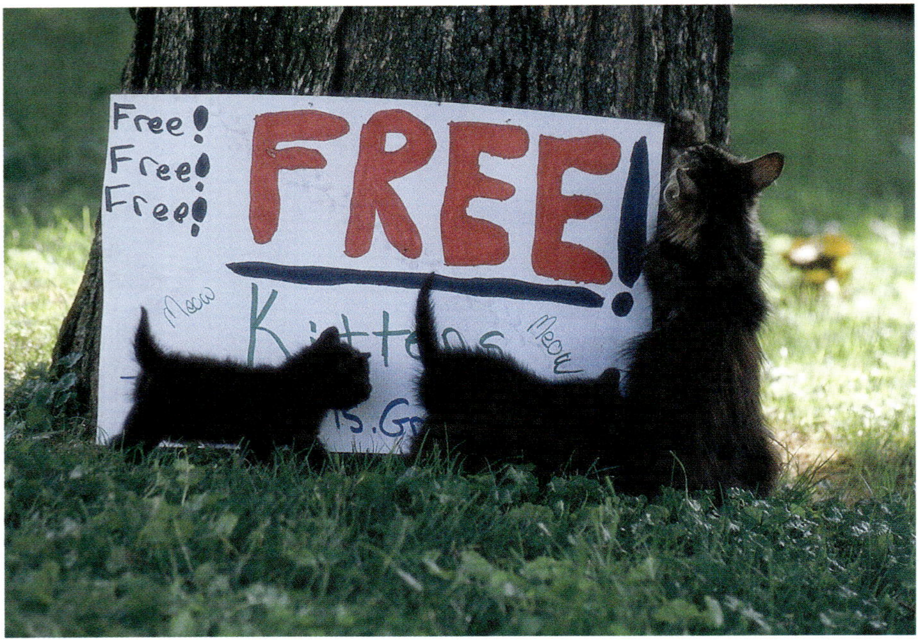

More kittens are born than homes can be found for.

tion and forage in dumpsters. Areas around restaurants, shopping centers, campgrounds, and schools contain feral cat colonies because cats can find available garbage to feed upon in these places.

Feral Cats

Throughout the United States, humanitarian people spend huge amounts of time and money bringing food to colonies of feral cats. These compassionate people only add to the problem since more cats survive and reproduce.

Organizations such as the *Alley Cat Allies* in Maryland and the *Feral Cat Coalition of Portland* in Oregon

Studies have shown that wild cats kill very few healthy birds. Birds are much harder to catch than roadkill, garbage, or even mice. Although the native songbird population is undoubtedly on the decline, feral cats are not to blame. Birds' habitats—the areas they require for nesting and feeding—are being destroyed at an astounding rate by human development. Unless this trend is reversed or modified, birds will soon have few places to live and nest. The depletion of the small bird population is not caused by feral cats.

No cat should be abandoned.

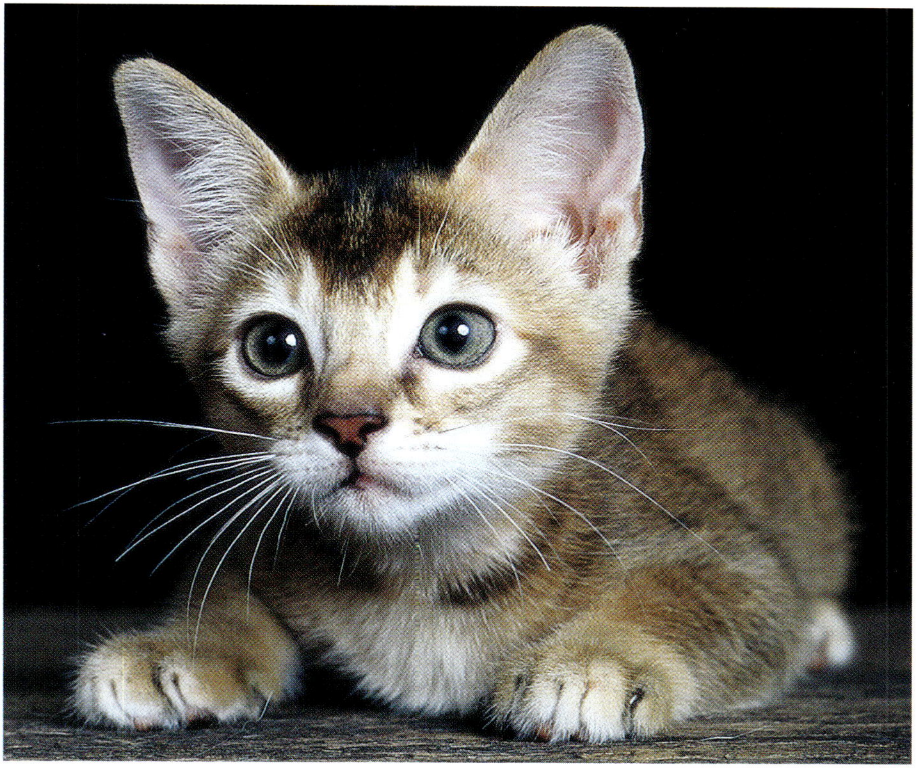

have formed in an attempt to stabilize the feral cat population. These groups have instituted programs to trap, vaccinate, alter, and release feral cats. Evidence shows that these efforts have little effect on reducing the numbers of cats in feral colonies. Some cats avoid the traps and continue to reproduce. New homeless cats join feral colonies where food is available.

The American Veterinary Medical Association supports actions to eliminate the problem of unwanted cats. The association recommends licensing and rabies vaccination requirements for cats. It encourages permanent identification and sterilization of all cats. It also suggests the removal of feral cats that are not in "managed colonies."

Taking Responsibility

An old Native American proverb says that someone who saves another person's life is forever responsible for the person saved. Kittens are not people, but the principle is the same. If you do not accept

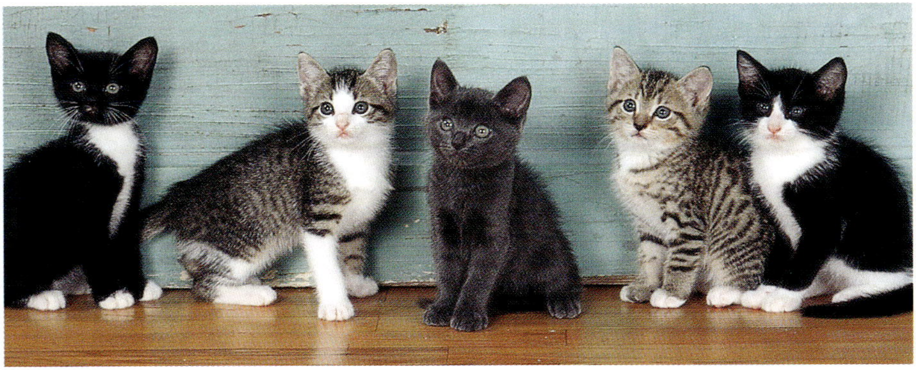

They are all beautiful and deserving of a loving home.

the challenge of raising orphaned kittens by hand, they would certainly die. If you are not willing to accept responsibility for your kittens' future, their fate may be worse than if they had died in infancy. They may have a short, painful life of starvation, cold, danger, and disease.

You need not plan to keep every kitten you hand-raise for your own pet. However, before you undertake the hand-raising of orphaned kittens, consider if you will be able to find real homes for them when the kittens are weaned.

Don't Add to Cat Overpopulation

- Can you find owners who will have the kittens neutered or spayed?
- Will their new owners have the kittens vaccinated? Will they feed the kittens properly?
- Are the new owners responsible people? Will they instead tire of the kittens and abandon them if they become a trouble or expense?

Do not go to the trouble of raising kittens by hand only to permit them to become some of the 60 million feral cats or the nine million cats euthanized at shelters every year. The population explosion among feral cats only produces more kittens to starve, freeze, and die. If you cannot find responsible homes for them, do not allow them to live for a short while only to die in misery. Plan ahead for the future of those little lives you work hard to save.

Glossary

Please note that the following definitions set forth the meanings of these terms as they are used specifically in this text. They are not intended to be complete definitions.

agalactia: without milk.
alter: to remove the reproductive organs of either sex surgically.
antibodies: proteins present in the blood that protect against disease.
ascarids: roundworms; the species *Toxocara cati* or *T. canis* in the cat.
aspiration pneumonia: pneumonia caused by breathing in foreign material.
ataxic: staggering; uncoordinated.
castrate: to remove the testicles surgically.
cat scratch disease: a bacterial disease caused by *Bartonella henselae*.
cerebellum: the portion of the brain that regulates the coordination of movements.
cerebrum: the part of the brain involved with consciousness.
coccidia: one-celled parasitic organisms.
colostrum: the first milk produced by a mother animal immediately after parturition.
congenital: present at birth.
contagious: transmissible from one animal to another.
cyst: a walled-off structure; in this text, a structure that contains an immature parasite.
definitive (final) host: the host in which a parasite lives in the last stage of its life cycle.
dystocia: difficult or impossible birth process.
esophagus: the tube through which an animal swallows food into its stomach.
estrus: the period in which a female animal will accept mating and will become pregnant.
euthanasia: *good death;* mercy killing.
external parasite: a parasite that lives on the body of a host.
feeding tube: a tube through which an animal receives nutrients.
feral: wild, reverting to a wild state.
fungus spore: the reproductive body of a fungus organism.
genetic: transmitted through the genes, inherited from one or both parents.
gestation: the period from impregnation to birth.
heartworm: a disease caused by the parasite *Dirofilaria immitis.*
host: the animal upon which a parasite lives.
host specific: a parasite that can live on only one species of host.
hydrocephalus: abnormal fluid in the cranial cavity.
hypocalcemia: insufficient amount of calcium in the body.

hypoplasia: underdevelopment, undersized.

incubation period: the period of time between infection and the appearance of a disease.

inherited: transmitted to offspring by one or both parents; genetic.

intermediate host: an animal in which a parasite lives in the second stage of its life cycle.

internal parasite: a parasite that lives entirely inside its host.

lactation: giving milk.

lactose: milk sugar.

larvae: the immature form of many animals; in this text, of parasites.

lesions: sores or wounds.

mastitis: an inflammation of the mammary glands.

microfilaria: the larval form of heartworm.

migrate: to travel.

mite: a parasite that causes skin disease; *Otodectes cynotis* are ear mites of cats.

nasogastric tube: a tube designed to be passed through the nose of a human infant.

neuter: to remove the reproductive organs, usually of the male.

oocysts, ova: two terms for eggs.

parasite: an organism that lives upon another animal.

parturition: the birth process.

perinatal: *around birth,* the period just before and just after birth.

placenta: the birth tissues.

polydactyl: having extra toes.

polyestrous: having several heat periods.

prepubertal: before puberty; before sexual maturity.

protozoa: one-celled organisms, some of which are parasitic.

puberty: the period of sexual maturity.

purulent: having a discharge of pus.

ringworm: a skin disease often caused by *Microsporum canis.*

roundworm: a common internal parasite.

scolex: the head of a tapeworm.

seasonally polyestrous: having many heat periods during one season of the year.

sibling: a brother or sister; a littermate.

spay: to remove the reproductive organs of the female surgically.

stomach tube: a tube passed into the stomach of an animal.

teratogen: a substance that can cause birth defects.

Toxacaral larval migrans: the medical condition in which the larvae of roundworms migrate through an animal's or a human's body.

toxin: a poison.

toxoplasmosis: a disease caused by *Toxoplasma gondii.*

trachea: the windpipe.

vermifuge: a medication that acts against internal parasites.

wean: to become able to eat solid food.

zoonosis (plural, zoonoses): a disease that can affect both animals and humans.

Useful Addresses and Literature

Books

Bulard-Cordeau, Brigitte, *Kittens,* Barron's Educational Series, Hauppauge, NY, 1997.

Cutts, Paddy, *The Complete Cat Book,* Smithmark, New York, NY, 1995.

Debietto, James, *Practical Kitten Care,* Howell Book House, New York, NY, 1996.

Evans, Mark, *The Complete Guide to Kitten Care,* Howell Book House, New York, NY, 1997.

Hurley, W. L., *Milk Composition,* University of Illinois, Urbana-Champaign, IL, 1997, http://classes.aces.uiue.edu/AnSci308/milkcomp.html

Pratt, Paul W., *Feline Medicine*, 1st Edition, American Veterinary Publications, Goleta, CA, 1983.

Maggitti, Phil, *Before You Buy That Kitten,* Barron's Educational Series, Hauppauge, NY, 1995.

Rice, Dan, *The Well-Mannered Cat,* Barron's Educational Series, Hauppauge, NY, 1998.

Rutherford, Alice, *The Readers' Digest Illustrated Book of Cats,* Readers' Digest Books, Montreal, Quebec, 1992.

Siegal, Mordecai, (Ed.), *The Cornell Book of Cats,* Villard Books, New York, NY, 1989.

Taylor, David, *The Ultimate Cat Book,* Simon and Schuster, New York, NY, 1989.

U.S. Pet Ownership & Demographics Sourcebook, The American Veterinary Medical Association, Schaumburg, IL, 1997.

Zoonosis Update, Second Edition, Journal of the American Veterinary Medical Association, Schaumburg, IL, 1995.

Sources of Equipment and Supplies

Local suppliers are the fastest sources of equipment and milk replacement formulas. Ask your veterinarian, or check your telephone book yellow pages under "Pet Supplies" or "Feed Stores."

These companies manufacture milk replacement formulas and equipment designed especially for kittens:

Farnum Companies, Inc.
301 W. Osborn Road
Phoenix, AZ 85013-3928
1-800-825-2555

Just Born milk replacement for kittens
Just Born hand-feeding kits and nursing bottles

Pet-Ag, Inc.
30 W. 43R, Rt. 20
Elgin, IL 60120
1-800-323-0877

KMR milk replacement for kittens
Kitten weaning formula
Esbilac nursing kits

Megadyne Products, Inc.
1227 S. Sheridan
Tulsa, OK 74112
1-800-MEGAPET

MegaDyne bottles and nipples

These are only some of the catalog sources of products and equipment:

Drs. Foster and Smith, Inc.
2253 Air Park Road, P.O. Box 100
Rhinelander, WI 54501-0100
1-800-826-7206

Jeffers Pet Catalog
P.O. Box 100
Dothan, AL 36302-0100
1-800-533-3377

New England Serum Company
P.O. Box 128
Topsfield, MA 01983-0228

Omaha Vaccine Company
P.O. Box 7228
Omaha, NE 68107
1-800-242-9447

Obtain a catalog and other information by calling any of the toll-free numbers listed above.

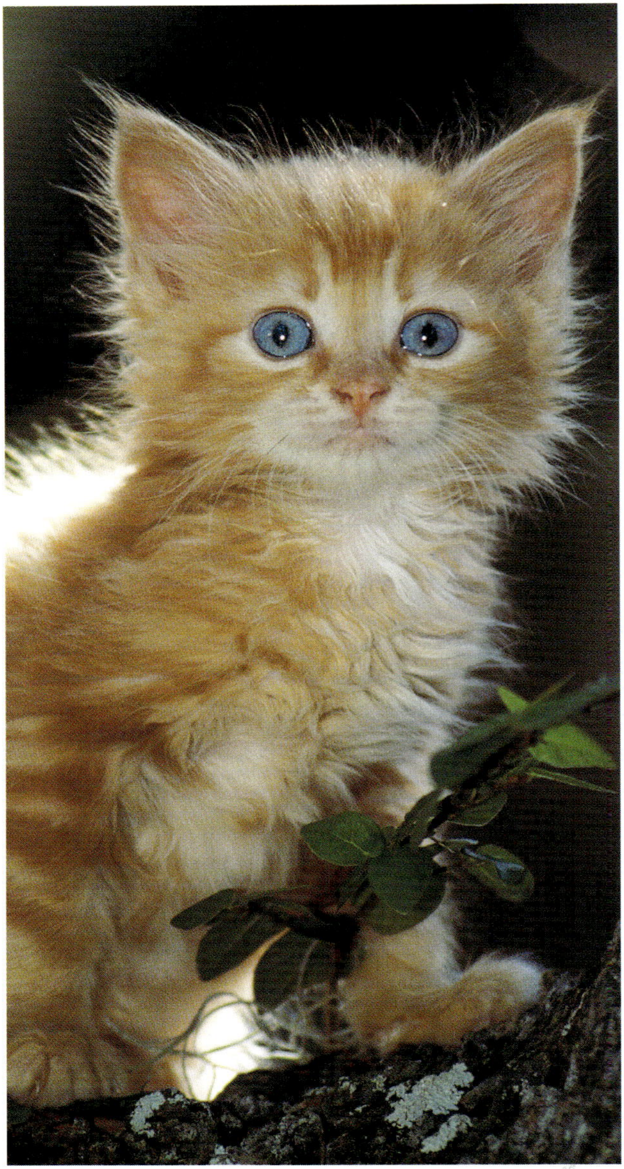

Index